NHS Audit Committee Handbook

Contents

Foreword and Introduction		4
Acknowledgements		5
Chapter 1:	Why the Governing Body Needs an Audit Committee	6
1.1	Why a Governing Body Has an Audit Committee – the Statutory Basis	6
1.2	What Does the Audit Committee do to Support the Governing Body?	6
	1.2.1 Assurance framework	8
	1.2.2 Disclosure statements	8
1.3	What Does the Audit Committee NOT do for the Governing Body?	9
1.4	What Authority Should the Governing Body Ensure that the Audit Committee Has?	9
1.5	What Relationship Does the Audit Committee Have with Auditors?	10
1.6	How Does the Audit Committee Report to the Governing Body?	10
Chapter 2:	How to Set Up and Support an Audit Committee	11
2.1	How Many Members Should an Audit Committee Have?	11
2.2	Who are the Members of the Audit Committee?	11
2.3	What Characteristics Should Audit Committee Members Possess?	12
2.4	What Makes a Meeting Quorate?	13
2.5	What are the Membership Terms?	13
2.6	How are Conflicts of Interest Handled?	13
2.7	Who Else Attends Audit Committee Meetings?	14
2.8	Who Chairs the Audit Committee?	14
2.9	What are the Training Needs of Audit Committee Members?	15
2.10	How Frequently Should the Audit Committee Meet?	16
2.11	What Administrative Support Should the Committee Expect?	16
2.12	How Should the Committee Assess its Own Performance?	17
2.13	What are the Implications of Collaborative Audit Committee Arrangements?	18
Chapter 3:	The Audit Committee and the Framework of Assurance	19
3.1	How Should the Audit Committee Focus its Work?	19
3.2	How Does the Committee Use and Support the Assurance Framework?	19
3.3	Assessing Risk	19
3.4	Reviewing the Assurance Framework's Format and Development	21
3.5	Reviewing the Strategic Objectives in the Assurance Framework	21
3.6	Assessing the Controls in the Assurance Framework	22
3.7	Reviewing the Assurances in the Assurance Framework	23

	3.8	Assurance Mapping	25
	3.9	Underlying Data	25
	3.10	Reviewing the Results of Assurances	26
	3.11	The Assurance Framework and Financial Control	26
	3.12	The Assurance Framework and Clinical Governance	27
	3.13	Clinical Risks Arising from Financial Pressures	28
	3.14	What Other Assurances Should be Sought?	28

Chapter 4: The Work of an Audit Committee — 30
- 4.1 How Does the Committee Work in Practice? — 30
- 4.2 How Does the Committee Review the Annual Report and Accounts? — 30
- 4.3 How Does the Committee Review the Annual Governance Statement? — 31
- 4.4 How Does the Committee Review Evidence Relating to the Organisation's Continuing 'Fitness to Function'? — 32
- 4.5 How Does the Committee Review the Quality Accounts? — 33
- 4.6 How Should the Committee Report During the Year? — 33
- 4.7 How Should the Committee Report at Year End? — 34

Chapter 5: Working with Other Committees and Auditors — 36
- 5.1 How Should the Audit Committee Relate to Other Committees? — 36
- 5.2 How do the Auditors Support the Audit Committee's Work? — 37
  - 5.2.1 Who are the internal auditors? — 37
  - 5.2.2 Who are the external auditors? — 37
  - 5.2.3 Who are the clinical auditors? — 38
- 5.3 How Does Internal Audit Support the Audit Committee's Work? — 38
  - 5.3.1 What does internal audit do? — 38
  - 5.3.2 The status of internal audit — 39
  - 5.3.3 How should the committee review the internal audit plan? — 40
  - 5.3.4 How should the committee review internal audit assignment reports? — 43
  - 5.3.5 How should the committee review the Head of Internal Audit's annual opinion? — 44
  - 5.3.6 How should the committee review the effectiveness of internal audit? — 45
  - 5.3.7 What is the committee's role in relation to third party assurances and hosted bodies and how does internal audit fit in? — 45
- 5.4 How Does External Audit Support the Audit Committee's Work? — 46
  - 5.4.1 What does external audit do? — 46
  - 5.4.2 The status of external audit — 46
  - 5.4.3 How should the committee review the external audit strategy and plan? — 47
  - 5.4.4 How should the committee deal with non-audit services? — 48
  - 5.4.5 How should the committee review external audit assignment reports? — 49
  - 5.4.6 How should the committee review external auditors' mandatory reports? — 50
- 5.5 How Does Clinical Audit Support the Audit Committee's Work? — 51

	5.6	How Does Counter (or Anti-) Fraud Activity Support the Audit Committee's Work?	53
	5.7	What is the Audit Committee's Role in Relation to Whistle Blowing?	54
	5.8	What is the Value of Private Discussions with the Auditors?	54

Appendix A: Example Terms of Reference   56

Appendix B: Example Agenda and Timetable   62

Appendix C: Self-assessment Checklists   64

Appendix D: Internal Audit Coverage   73

Appendix E: References and Further Reading   78

Foreword and Introduction

Welcome to the 2014 version of the *NHS Audit Committee Handbook* which is designed to help NHS governing bodies and audit committees as they review and continually re-assess their system of governance, risk management and control to ensure that it remains effective and 'fit for purpose' across all that an organisation does. It has been developed by the HFMA's Governance and Audit Committee to provide a self-contained source of guidance for all members of audit committees and will also be of interest to those who serve on governing bodies.

The Handbook replaces the 2011 edition and, although it has been fully updated to take account of the many changes that the NHS has seen since then, the underlying principles, structure and content of the Handbook will be familiar to many. In particular, it continues to provide audit committee members with a succinct summary of what is expected from them and a series of practical tips and pointers to help them put the theory into practice.

In response to comments from users of the Handbook, we have also:

- Compared our guidance with other relevant documents including the *UK Corporate Governance Code*; the Financial Reporting Council's *Guidance on Audit Committees*; the Treasury's *Audit and Risk Assurance Committee Handbook*; Monitor's *Code of Governance* and *Audit Code* and the *NHS Wales Audit Committee Handbook*
- Reduced the number of appendices with relevant references included in the main body of the guidance.

As with earlier versions, this Handbook applies to NHS organisations in England – however, the principles and much of the practical guidance is broadly relevant across the rest of the UK. In terms of its content, the Handbook starts by explaining why governing bodies need audit committees and how they provide support in fulfilling statutory duties and organisational objectives. It then looks at how audit committees should be set up before moving on to focus in detail on what they do and how they work with others. Practical examples and case studies are included throughout to bring the theory to life and cross references to further sources of guidance are include both within the text and as an appendix.

Audit committees and their members continue to play a crucial role in the governance of every NHS organisation and members must take seriously their responsibility for scrutinising the risks and controls affecting every aspect of the business – not just in the finance and financial management sphere. We hope that you find this Handbook of real practical benefit as you carry out this demanding role.

If you have any comments or suggestions about how we could develop the Handbook in future, please let us know via publications@hfma.org.uk

Kevin Stringer
Chair, HFMA Governance and Audit Committee

Acknowledgements

This Handbook was developed by the HFMA's Governance and Audit Committee. The HFMA is grateful to all those who attend the committee's meetings (either as full members or guests) and their employing organisations for their help and support. In particular we would like to thank:

Kevin Stringer (Chair of the committee), Chief Financial Officer, The Royal Wolverhampton Hospitals NHS Trust
Francesca Annetta, Head of Finance, Care Quality Commission
Laura Brackwell, National Audit Office
Rod Barnes, Executive Director of Finance and Performance, Yorkshire Ambulance Service NHS Trust
Steve Connor, Deputy Director, Mersey Internal Audit Agency
Derek Corbett, Director of Audit, Barts and The London NHS Trust
Paul Dudfield, Consortium Director, CW Audit Services
David Gregory, Head of Internal Audit, Leeds Teaching Hospitals NHS Trust
Andrew Kendrick, Technical Manager, Audit Commission
Jenny McCall, Director of Audit, Audit South West
David Milner, Associate Manager (Health), Public Sector Consultants
Glen Palethorpe, Partner, Risk Advisory, Baker Tilley
Val Peacock, Head of Audit, City Hospitals Sunderland NHS Foundation Trust
Antony Rodden, Director, Shared Services Task Force
Phil Rule, Director, PHP Consulting Limited
Phil Sharman, Director of Audit and Assurance, NHS Wales Shared Services Partnership
Pat Shroff, Independent Consultant
Michael Townsend, Regional Managing Director, TIAA
Paul Traynor, Director of Finance, East and North Hertfordshire NHS Trust
Joanna Watson, Senior Manager, PriceWaterhouseCoopers
Clare Winch, Head of Assurance, Oxford University Hospitals NHS Trust
Lynn Wilson, Director of Performance, TIAA
John Yarnold, Independent Consultant, Mount Vernon Consulting.

The HFMA is also grateful to all those who commented on drafts of the Handbook.

The Handbook was edited by Anna Green, Technical Editor, HFMA.

Chapter 1: Why the Governing Body Needs an Audit Committee

> This chapter explains that every governing body/board[1] is required to have an audit committee to support them in fulfilling their statutory and organisational objectives. It summarises the key ways in which audit committees provide this support.

1.1 Why a Governing Body Has an Audit Committee – the Statutory Basis

Every NHS organisation is required to have an audit committee that reports to its governing body.[2] The formal requirements to have an audit committee are set out in different documents, depending on the organisation:

- For clinical commissioning groups (CCGs), s14M of of the *NHS Act 2006* (inserted by s25 of the *2012 Act*) and NHS England's *Model Constitution Framework* (section 6.6.3)
- For foundation trusts (FTs), Monitor's *NHS Foundation Trust Code of Governance*
- For non-foundation NHS trusts, the NHS Trust Development Authority's *Code of Conduct and Accountability*.[3]

1.2 What Does the Audit Committee do to Support the Governing Body?

NHS governing body members have a daunting task in overseeing some of the largest and most complex organisations in the country. To fulfil this role it is the governing body's responsibility to put in place governance structures and processes to:

- Ensure that the organisation operates effectively and meets its statutory and strategic objectives
- Provide it (i.e. the governing body) with assurance[4] that this is the case.

However, even the best structures and processes can let down an organisation if they (and the assurances they provide) are not operated with sufficient rigour – this is where audit

---

[1] For many organisations the governing body is known as the board. In foundation trusts there is also a Council of Governors. To avoid repetition, we have used the generic term 'governing body' throughout this Handbook.

[2] All NHS bodies are required to have a governing body (or board) which comprises both executive and non-executive directors (NEDs)/lay members. This governing body is separate from the day-to-day management structure. The exact structure of each governing body is different for each type of NHS body and is set out in legislation and associated regulations. For non-foundation NHS trusts the relevant legislation is regulations 2 and 4 of the *1990 Trust Membership and Procedure Regulations (SI 1990/2024)*. For FTs, there is a board (or 'council') of governors and a board of directors as required in schedule 7 to the *NHS Act 2006*. For clinical commissioning groups (CCGs), the requirement to have a governing body (that has its functions delegated to it by the CCG 'council of members' on which all the CCG's constituent GP practices are represented, is set out in s14L of the *NHS Act 2006* (inserted by s25 of the 2012 Act) and the associated regulations (SI 2012/1631).

[3] *Code of Conduct and Accountability*, NHS Trust Development Authority, 2013: www.ntda.nhs.uk/wp-content/uploads/2013/04/CODE-OF-CONDUCT-AND-ACCOUNTABILITY-FOR-NHS-BOARDS.pdf

[4] Assurance is defined by the Treasury in *The Orange Book: Management of Risk – Principles and Concepts* as 'an evaluated opinion, based on evidence gained from review, on the organisation's risk management and internal control framework'.

committees play a key role in supporting the governing body by critically reviewing and reporting on the relevance and robustness of the governance structures and assurance processes on which the governing body places reliance. In particular, this requires the audit committee to understand and scrutinise the organisation's overarching framework of governance, risk and control. At the corporate level this includes risk management and performance management systems underpinned by the assurance framework.[5] This framework sets out the organisation's 'mission critical' objectives and identifies the key risks that could prevent their achievement. In effect, it is the 'lens' through which the governing body examines the assurances it requires to discharge its duties.

The audit committee also supports the governing body by:

- Obtaining assurances about controls and whether they are working as they should
- Seeking assurances about the underlying data (upon which assurances are based) to ensure that it is robust, reliable and accurate
- Challenging poor and/or unreliable sources of assurance
- Challenging relevant managers when controls are not working or data is unreliable.

Audit committees also continue to play a key role in scrutinising financial control matters and reporting on them to the governing body. However, it is important to recognise that their focus extends across **all** of an organisation's activities. This wider focus is particularly marked in the NHS, where governing bodies have to meet a broad range of stakeholder requirements and achieve an overall objective of delivering high quality healthcare. A number of governance lapses over recent years have underlined the need for governance policies, procedures and structures that:

- Put the interests of patients at the heart of what an organisation does
- Recognise the critical importance of quality
- Are comprehensive
- Work in practice, not just on paper.

> **Lessons from Governance Failings at Mid-Staffordshire NHS Foundation Trust**
>
> The Healthcare Commission's 2009 investigation into Mid-Staffordshire NHS Foundation Trust (where multiple management failures led to higher mortality rates), found that the Trust, which was seeking to make financial savings in order to apply for foundation trust status, appeared to 'have lost sight of its real priorities'.
>
> The 2010 report by Robert Francis QC revealed that deficiencies in staffing and governance extended over a period of more than 5 years and yet remained un-remedied by those responsible. His 2013 report went further and found that the Trust had failed to listen to patients' concerns, correct deficiencies and tackle an 'insidious negative culture' that tolerated poor standards and clinical disengagement from managerial and leadership responsibilities. The report concluded that 'this failure was in part the consequence of allowing a focus on reaching national access targets, achieving financial balance and seeking foundation trust status at the cost of delivering acceptable standards of care.'

---

[5] This Handbook uses the generic term 'assurance framework' throughout. However, some organisations use the term 'board (or governing body) assurance framework'.

As far as the governing body is concerned there are two key areas on which it should look to the audit committee for assurance: the assurance framework itself and the public disclosure statements that flow from the assurance processes.

1.2.1 Assurance framework

Given that governing bodies rely on an assurance framework to monitor strategic objectives and identify significant inherent risks, the audit committee's primary role is to look behind it to provide assurance that the framework itself is valid and suitable for the governing body's requirements. Through its work, the audit committee can review whether:

- The format of the assurance framework is appropriate for the organisation
- The way in which the framework is developed is robust and relevant
- The objectives in the framework reflect the governing body's priorities and that both the objectives and priorities are well defined, agreed and recorded
- The key risks are identified and linked to objectives
- The controls in place are sound and complete
- The assurances are reliable and of good quality with all key sources identified
- The underlying data on which assurances are based is reliable, accurate and timely
- There are actions in place to address gaps in control and/or assurance and that they are implemented in line with agreed timescales.

In this way the audit committee provides valuable assurances to the governing body that the organisation has sufficient controls in place to manage the significant risks to achieving its strategic objectives and that these controls are operating effectively. The committee also alerts the governing body to any areas where controls are lacking or not operating as they should and where mitigating actions are needed. This activity is described in more detail in chapter 3.

1.2.2 Disclosure statements

The audit committee also has a pivotal role to play in reviewing the disclosure statements that flow from the organisation's assurance processes prior to their submission to the full governing body. In particular these comprise:

- The annual report and accounts
- The annual quality account/report
- The annual governance statement (informed by the annual Head of Internal Audit Opinion)
- The evidence required to demonstrate (on an on-going basis) that fitness to be registered with the Care Quality Commission is maintained and that the organisation is fulfilling the terms of Monitor's license
- In the case of clinical commissioning groups, evidence to show that the terms of authorisation are being met on an ongoing basis
- Other statements such as returns required by NHS England, the NHS Trust Development Authority (NHS TDA), Monitor and the Care Quality Commission.

The focus for the audit committee is on seeking assurances about the rigour of the processes followed in preparing the statements and the quality of the underlying data upon which they are based. The quality and reliability of the data used is of particular importance as the audit committee must feel confident that the disclosures are well founded if it is to provide assurances to the governing body. This activity is described in more detail in chapter 4.

1.3 What Does the Audit Committee NOT do for the Governing Body?

To establish and cement its role, it is important that the audit committee has no executive responsibilities and does not take on any roles or duties that are not those of an audit committee. In particular, it is **not** the job of the audit committee to establish and maintain processes for governance. This is the responsibility of the organisation's executive directors and the Accountable (or Accounting) Officer (i.e. the organisation's Chief Officer – usually the Chief Executive).[6]

It is also important that:

- The audit committee is neither a finance committee nor an investment committee, with responsibility for regular review and approval of financial reports or investment proposals
- The audit committee does not manage the risk agenda on a day-to-day basis – the organisation will have an executive structure for this (see sections 3.3 and 5.1).

1.4 What Authority Should the Governing Body Ensure that the Audit Committee Has?

The audit committee must be invested with sufficient authority to act with independence. It should be constituted as a committee of the governing body and the terms of reference should be agreed by the governing body and set out in its minutes. The terms of reference should also be available publicly.[7] Example terms of reference are included at Appendix A.

The audit committee should have explicit authority to receive full access to information (including from any external organisations providing services to the organisation – for example a commissioning support unit) and the ability to investigate any matters within its terms of reference, including the right to independent professional advice. The committee should also be empowered to require any member of staff of the organisation to report to it on the risks and controls that they are responsible for, either via a written report or attendance at a meeting.

In every organisation it is essential that a senior member of staff (for example, the organisation's secretary or governance lead) is responsible for ensuring that the committee receives the resources and support that it needs to fulfil its role.

---

[6] Two terms are used for the same role to distinguish between an Accounting Officer (for example in a foundation trust) who is directly accountable to Parliament (via the Public Accounts Committee) and an Accountable Officer (for example, in a clinical commissioning group or non-foundation NHS trust) who is responsible to an Accounting Officer of a government department who is in turn accountable to Parliament.

[7] For FTs, the requirement to make the terms of reference publicly available is set out in provision C.3.2 of Monitor's *Code of Governance*.

1.5 What Relationship Does the Audit Committee Have with Auditors?

It is important that the governing body understands the relationship between its audit committee and the organisation's internal and external auditors. The key point is that auditors are central to the audit committee's role as they can provide both assurance and insight into the management arrangements within the organisation. Indeed, the Head of Internal Audit is required to provide the audit committee with an annual opinion on the overall adequacy and effectiveness of the organisation's risk management, control and governance processes to underpin and support the annual governance statement.

Increasingly, and to support their wider role, audit committees are also seeking assurances from (and working with) clinical auditors. These relationships are explored more fully in chapter 5, which also refers to the audit committee's role in monitoring the quality of internal and external auditors and, in certain circumstances, playing a part in their appointment.

1.6 How Does the Audit Committee Report to the Governing Body?

Audit committee meetings and their minutes should be formal. The minutes should be presented at the next governing body meeting and these should be made public, as far as possible. It is good practice to include with the minutes a summary report highlighting any key issues or advice.

The governing body should agree with the audit committee what assurances it requires and when it needs to receive them. This point was emphasised in the Audit Commission's 2009 report *Taking it on Trust* which stated:

> 'The governing body needs to agree with the audit committee what assurances it requires and when, to feed its annual business cycle. In order to meet these expectations the audit committee needs a clear view of its programme across the year. In reality, these expectations are likely to relate to certifications that the governing body must make, including returns to Monitor and the Care Quality Commission.... However, increasingly, this might also involve assurances over the control of major projects or business processes.'

In practice, this means that, in addition to its minutes, the audit committee should provide the governing body with formal reports of its work, the assurances that have been received and validated and any that are missing, along with details of how such gaps are to be addressed. Reports may also include details of unexpected risks or problems that emerge (for example, as a result of whistle blowing). In such instances, the committee will need to ensure that arrangements are in place to allow issues to be properly and thoroughly investigated with a way forward identified and reported to the governing body when appropriate.

The governing body should also receive an annual summary report from the audit committee but will be helped in its own work if the committee provides one or more interim reports on matters relevant to, or specified by, the governing body. This is discussed in more detail in chapter 4.

Chapter 2: How to Set Up and Support an Audit Committee

> This chapter focuses on how audit committees are constituted and how they operate in practice. It also looks at the implications of collaborative arrangements that may exist in clinical commissioning groups and at the importance of reviewing the committee's own effectiveness via regular self-assessments.

2.1 How Many Members Should an Audit Committee Have?

The Treasury's guidance as set out in its *Audit and Risk Assurance Committee Handbook* should be followed – this states that audit committees should comprise at least three non-executive directors (or lay members).[1]

2.2 Who are the Members of the Audit Committee?

The distinctive characteristic of the audit committee is that it comprises independent, objective non-executive directors (NEDs) or lay members[2] who are appointed by the organisation's governing body. In other words, audit committee members should satisfy the governing body's definition of 'independence' and:

- **Not** be employed by the organisation (other than in their capacity as members of the audit committee)
- **Not** claim a significant proportion of their 'trading income'[3] from the organisation.

In foundation trusts (FTs), Monitor's *Code of Governance* (provision C.3.1) states that 'the board of directors should establish an audit committee composed of at least three members who are **all** independent non-executive directors'. For non-foundation trusts and clinical commissioning groups, the Department of Health's 2013 consultation paper *Health Service Bodies Audit Committees*[4] proposed that the committee should 'normally, wholly or mainly, comprise of independent non-executive members of the governing board' and that it must have a majority of independent non-executive members.

---

[1] This is in line with the requirement set out in the FRC's 2012 *UK Corporate Governance Code* which requires boards in the private sector to establish an audit committee of at least three, or in the case of smaller companies, two independent non-executive directors. Monitor's *Code of Governance* builds on the UK Code and requires foundation trusts to establish an audit committee composed of NEDs which should include at least three independent NEDs.

[2] For clinical commissioning groups, schedule 2, paragraph 7 (3) of the *Health and Social Care Act 2012* says that 'Arrangements.... **may** include provision for the audit committee to include individuals who are not members of the governing body.' However, NHS England's *Model Constitution Framework* for CCGs recommends that they should follow the *NHS Audit Committee Handbook*.

[3] Trading income refers to income received from the organisation for services provided. This does not include a fee or expenses that may be received for serving as a NED or lay member.

[4] At the time of writing (April 2013), the Department's guidance had not been finalised. For the latest position go to: https://www.gov.uk/government/consultations/new-requirements-for-nhs-audit-committees

This condition of membership provides the basis for the committee to operate independently of any executive management processes and to apply an objective approach in the conduct of its business.

The governing body is responsible for determining whether or not a prospective member of the audit committee is independent but guidance documents issued by the Department of Health[5] and Monitor[6] identify issues that need to be taken into account when doing this.

It is also important that the Chair of the organisation itself should not be a member of the audit committee and should not normally attend meetings.

Membership of the audit committee should be disclosed in the organisation's annual report.

2.3 What Characteristics Should Audit Committee Members Possess?

Given the importance and complexity of the audit committee's work, it is essential that at least one member has recent relevant financial experience.[7] It is also advantageous for members to have relevant skills or experience – for example, in the clinical, financial or risk management fields. Membership is also best suited to non-executives/lay members who have a background of serving on equivalent committees in other organisations. If this is not possible, the committee's Chair should ensure that members receive the training and support that they need to be effective in their role. Audit committee members should also be told what is expected of them (including the likely time commitment) and receive suitable induction and training to meet their needs (see section 2.9).

As well as relevant skills and experience, audit committee members should be courteous in their dealings and adhere to the *Seven Principles of Public Life* that were set out by the Nolan Committee in 1995.

> **The Principles of Public Life**
>
> - **Selflessness** – holders of public office should take decisions solely in terms of the public interest. They should not do so in order to gain financial or other material benefits for themselves, their family, or their friends

---

[5] At the time of writing (April 2013), the Department's guidance had not been finalised: refer to its website for the latest position:
https://www.gov.uk/government/consultations/new-requirements-for-nhs-audit-committees

[6] In FTs, the board of directors is responsible for determining whether a non-executive director is independent in line with the criteria set out in provision B.1.1 of the *NHS Foundation Trust Code of Governance* issued by Monitor in 2013.

[7] For CCGs, NHS England stipulates (in section 6.6.2d of the *Model Constitution Framework*) that the lay member for governance (who is required to chair a CCG's audit committee) must have qualifications, expertise or experience that enables her/him to express informed views about financial management. The Treasury's *Audit and Risk Assurance Committee Handbook* requires the audit committee chair to have 'relevant experience' and both the FRC's *UK Corporate Governance Code* and Monitor's *Code of Governance* (provision C.3.1) require the board to satisfy itself that at least one member has 'recent and relevant financial experience'.

- **Integrity** – holders of public office should not place themselves under any financial or other obligation to outside individuals or organisations that might influence them in the performance of their official duties
- **Objectivity** – in carrying out public business, including making public appointments, awarding contracts, or recommending individuals for rewards and benefits, holders of public office should make choices on merit
- **Accountability** – holders of public office are accountable for their decisions and actions to the public and must submit to whatever scrutiny is appropriate to their office
- **Openness** – holders of public office should be as open as possible about all the decisions and actions that they take. They should give reasons for their decisions and restrict information only when the wider public interest clearly demands it
- **Honesty** – holders of public office have a duty to declare any private interests relating to their public duties and to take steps to resolve any conflicts arising in a way that protects the public interest
- **Leadership** – holders of public office should promote and support these principles by leadership and example.

2.4 What Makes a Meeting Quorate?

It is important to have a clear policy on what constitutes a quorate meeting – in our view, this should be a minimum of two of the three independent non-executive/lay members of the audit committee who are also members of the organisation's governing body.

2.5 What are the Membership Terms?

The duration of appointments to the committee and the process and timescales for renewal is a matter for the governing body but should be made clear when membership begins. The policy adopted in this area is a matter of judgement for the organisation's governing body, but a balance needs to be struck between bringing in fresh perspectives and maintaining an experienced membership that has established effective relationships with those that attend the committee.

The Treasury's *Audit and Risk Assurance Committee Handbook* recommends that all committee members receive a formal letter of appointment covering key expectations and responsibilities.

2.6 How are Conflicts of Interest Handled?

Any potential conflicts of interest should be dealt with in accordance with existing codes of practice/policies that operate within the organisation. This will ensure consistency with the approach taken by the governing body and is likely to involve requiring every committee member to take personal responsibility for declaring potential conflicts and the committee Chair then determining an appropriate course of action – for example, asking the member to leave the meeting whilst a particular item is considered. If a conflict is likely to continue for some time, the member may be asked to stand down from the committee.

In some CCGs, it is possible that lay/independent members may be shared with another CCG audit committee. Where this is the case each audit committee Chair needs to ensure that there is:

- A formal declaration from each member about their other roles at the start of each meeting and that this is recorded in the minutes
- A written protocol setting out how conflicts of interest will be addressed and recorded.

2.7 Who Else Attends Audit Committee Meetings?

Although they should not be members of the audit committee, the Accountable/Accounting Officer and all other executive directors will attend whenever they are invited by the audit committee's Chair and, in particular, to provide assurances and explanations to the committee when it is discussing audit reports or other matters within their areas of responsibility. For example, as a minimum, the Accountable/Accounting Officer would be expected to be present when the committee considers the draft annual governance statement and the annual report and accounts.

It is for the audit committee Chair to plan the meetings and invite executive directors and other senior managers according to the requirements of each agenda. This will vary from meeting to meeting and will depend on whose area of responsibility an agenda item falls within. Directors/managers should be given sufficient warning that their presence is required so that they come fully prepared.

Representatives from internal and external audit, together with the senior member of staff responsible for the committee (this is likely to be the organisation's secretary or governance lead) and the Chief Finance Officer (CFO)[8] would normally be present at every audit committee meeting with the counter (or anti-) fraud specialist[9] attending a minimum of two committees per year.

2.8 Who Chairs the Audit Committee?

The selection of the Chair is a critical appointment for the organisation as the role's responsibilities differ from those of other non-executive directors/lay members. In most cases, the person appointed to this role will possess a prior understanding of finance and internal control or other relevant expertise such as risk management. In CCGs, NHS England guidance specifies that the lay member for governance should chair the audit committee[10] and that he or she must have qualifications, expertise or experience that enables them to express informed views about financial management.[11] Treasury guidance[12] also requires the audit committee

---

[8] We have used the generic term 'Chief Finance Officer' throughout this Handbook to stand for the most senior finance professional in an organisation – in practice, many organisations use the title Finance Director, Director of Finance or Chief Financial Officer.

[9] In some organisations the term 'anti-fraud' will be used instead of 'counter fraud' – to avoid repetition of both phrases, this Handbook uses counter fraud throughout.

[10] *CCG Governing Body Members: role outlines, attributes and skills*, NHS England, 2012.

[11] *NHS England Model Constitution Framework*, section 6.6.2d.

[12] *Audit and Risk Assurance Committee Handbook*, HM Treasury, 2013.

Chair to be a non-executive board (governing body) member with 'relevant experience' and includes a useful appendix on the role of the Chair with a focus on how to ensure that the committee is effective.

As mentioned above, the Chair of the organisation should not be a member of the audit committee.

> **Case Study – the Tasks of One Audit Committee Chair in a Foundation Trust**
> - Liaise with the trust secretary to plan and prepare the audit committee's work and papers (agendas/minutes/annual plan/annual report/terms of reference)
> - Invite executive directors and senior managers to attend according to the needs of each agenda
> - Review full internal and external audit reports (other audit committee members receive summaries prepared by the auditors of significant findings and recommendations)
> - Meet privately with internal and external auditors, the chief executive and CFO to discuss audit committee matters
> - Visit both internal audit and finance staff at least twice a year
> - Receive papers from the 'integrated governance committee'
> - Attend national/regional groups as appropriate
> - Report regularly to the governing body on audit committee activities
> - Report to the council of governors on relevant issues (for example, the re-appointment of external auditors).

2.9 What are the Training Needs of Audit Committee Members?

The committee should consider its own training needs so that members have the skills that will allow them to perform their role effectively. In particular, every member needs to have a basic understanding of finance and internal control. Some members will have this before they are appointed; others should be provided with suitable training at an early stage, as part of their induction. Training that will help develop audit committee members may include:

- Background to their role and what distinguishes it from that of other governing body members. This is likely to include exploring current trends in good governance (including clinical), risk management and assurance; the role of internal and external auditors; the role of local counter fraud specialists and how to improve audit committee effectiveness
- The issues an audit committee should focus on – for example, background and good practice in the oversight of the disclosure statements that the audit committee reviews and understanding the organisation's risk profile and control environment.

Opportunities arise from time to time for meetings of audit committee members, where they can share knowledge and experience and listen to expert speakers. Informal meetings of audit committee Chairs also provide a valuable opportunity to share knowledge and best practice. In addition literature and advice on audit committees is available, much of it online. Sources specific to the NHS include the Department of Health; NHS England; the NHS Trust Development Authority; Monitor; audit providers and professional associations such as the HFMA. Helpful guidance is also available from professional accountancy bodies and from risk management and audit organisations.

2.10 How Frequently Should the Audit Committee Meet?

The frequency of meetings should be driven by the nature and timing of the business to be considered, any complementary work conducted by other committees and any work that can be carried out between meetings. This all needs to be determined at the outset of the financial year so that the committee is not considering unnecessary issues, reacting to foreseeable events or commenting on matters that can no longer be influenced. Given the breadth of an NHS audit committee's remit and the need to retain a focused financial scrutiny role, we take the view that it is unlikely to be able to fulfil all of its responsibilities in fewer than five meetings a year[13] (this includes meetings planned for a specific purpose – for example, to consider the annual report and accounts).

Ultimately, this decision is one for the governing body and the committee to make with a view to ensuring that the committee meets its terms of reference. Reducing the other commitments of the committee's Chair, and perhaps other committee members, may create additional capacity to allow more frequent meetings, but this needs to be balanced with the need to understand in sufficient breadth the organisation's activities.

Appendix B provides an example audit committee timetable tracking key agenda items over the year – it assumes that five meetings are held.

2.11 What Administrative Support Should the Committee Expect?

As with any committee, effective work is best achieved if there is strong administrative support that allows the members of the committee to concentrate on their role in preparing for (and contributing to) the meeting. It is also important that all members of the committee attend regularly and participate actively and that the Chair is not too dominant.

For an audit committee to make effective use of its limited time it needs to have sufficient resources and in particular, the support of a strong secretary. This is an important role and is generally assumed by the organisation's secretary or governance lead. In any case, it should be carried out by a senior member of staff of the organisation so that the audit committee's influence continues to be felt between meetings. The Secretary should not be the CFO or the Head of Internal Audit or somebody reporting to either.

As mentioned in section 2.10 above, the timing of meetings is critical in helping the committee to discharge its various responsibilities and needs to be discussed with all the parties involved

---

[13] The Treasury says in its *Audit and Risk Assurance Committee Handbook* that committees need to meet 'at **least** four times a year'.

(including the Head of Internal Audit, the external auditors, the Accountable/Accounting Officer and the CFO) to ensure that key tasks, such as the approval of the annual report and accounts, are accommodated. The detailed planning of meetings is likely to be the responsibility of the secretary to the audit committee.

The example terms of reference in appendix A includes a section on the administrative support that the committee should expect to receive.

2.12 How Should the Committee Assess its Own Performance?

Audit committees should assess their own performance and effectiveness annually and report the results to the governing body. In framing this assessment, it is helpful to think in terms of a number of overarching key measures of success – for example:

- What difference has the committee made to the organisation's governance, risk and control environment?
- Did the committee encounter any 'surprises' during the year that it should have seen coming – for example, did the organisation receive any unexpected adverse inspection reports?
- Did the committee have to re-focus its planned activities during the year – if so was this a pro-active decision or for reactive reasons?

It is also helpful to seek the views of both internal and external auditors (and the local counter fraud specialist where relevant) about how they view the committee's effectiveness.

Appendix C includes two checklists that will help support this assessment – the first focuses on process issues (with simple yes/no answers) and can be completed by the committee's Chair and secretary. The second probes more deeply into how well the committee and its members feel they are performing. As with any self-assessment, it is important that committee members are constructively critical in their responses.

The committee should draw up its own plan for improvement as a result of the self-assessment, either in requesting training or development for members, or in changes to its processes and procedures.

> **Best Practice – Audit Committee Self-assessment**
>
> - Audit committee members should complete the agreed checklist and the results should be collated by someone independent of the members, such as the committee's secretary
> - The involvement of the auditors, either internal or external, may help in interpreting the questions or discussing best practice, given their likely experience with other audit committees
> - In areas of doubt, the committee may wish to look at other self-assessment checklists for audit committees, or ask for advice on best practice in other parts of the public and private sectors.

2.13 What are the Implications of Collaborative Audit Committee Arrangements?

In some CCGs, an audit committee may meet at the same time as another CCG audit committee. Whilst this approach clearly offers CCGs the potential for some efficiencies and sharing of knowledge and expertise at all levels, it is essential that each CCG can demonstrate that it is discharging its own statutory duties and that no conflicts of interest impair its independence. It must be borne in mind at all times that each CCG is a separate statutory body.

Where audit committees are operating in this way, they should therefore ensure that they have in place clear, agreed protocols defining their working arrangements and how the declaration and recording of any conflicts of interest is to be handled.

> **Good Practice for Collaborative Arrangements – How a CCG Can Ensure that its Own Audit Committee Discharges its Statutory Duties**
>
> Each CCG audit committee should have:
>
> - Its own Chair – where this is not feasible and the same person chairs more than one CCG audit committee, it must be clear which committee is being chaired when
> - Its own terms of reference (including protocols for working with other CCG audit committees where appropriate)
> - Its own agenda and minutes
> - Details about who its members are and their status (for example, whether or not they are voting members)
> - Separate attendance records for each meeting (for example, if members belong to only one committee is their attendance at the other committee's meeting noted?)
> - Details of how conflicts of interest are addressed and recorded
> - A formal declaration of members' other roles at the start of each meeting, recorded in the minutes
> - Separate reports to its own governing body
> - An assessment of its effectiveness, at least annually (see section 2.12 and Appendix C).

Chapter 3: The Audit Committee and the Framework of Assurance

> This chapter looks in detail at the audit committee's role in relation to the assurance framework and the underlying risk management system. It also considers the committee's focus on assurances relating to financial control and clinical governance.

3.1 How Should the Audit Committee Focus its Work?

We saw in chapter 1 that the assurance framework is the key source of evidence that links the organisation's 'mission critical' strategic objectives to risks, controls and assurances, and is the main tool that the governing body uses in discharging its overall responsibility for internal control. The primary role of the audit committee is to continually review the relevance and rigour of the assurance framework and the arrangements surrounding it. To this end the committee should use the framework both as the central tool for planning its work and as a key topic for its scrutiny. If it does this, the committee is able to provide the governing body with assurances about the content and operation of the framework.

3.2 How Does the Committee Use and Support the Assurance Framework?

The work of the audit committee is not to manage the process of populating the assurance framework or to become involved in the operational development of risk management processes, either at an overall level or for individual risks. These are the responsibility of the governing body supported by line management. The audit committee's role is to satisfy itself that the systems and processes in place are working as they should.

In particular, the committee should review the processes for developing the framework and its format to ensure that they remain relevant and effective for the organisation. In this way, the committee can provide assurance that the framework concentrates on the 'right' high risk areas – in other words, those areas where either the inherent risk is high and the level of dependence upon the operation of controls is critical, or where the residual risk is high and the situation needs monitoring.

3.3 Assessing Risk

For an organisation's assurance framework to be effective there must be a robust system in place for the identification, assessment and prioritisation of risk. All risks identified by an organisation should be scored using a system that enables them to be ranked in terms of their importance. This normally takes account of the likelihood of a risk occurring and the impact on the organisation if it does. Once risks have been ranked, a decision can be made as to whether they need to be mitigated or managed through the application of controls or avoided, transferred or accepted.

Good risk management encourages organisations to take well-managed risks that allow safe development, growth and change. However, as it is impossible to eliminate all risks, every organisation has to live with a degree of risk. It is for the governing body to decide the balance between the cost of mitigating risks, tolerating risks and accepting the risk which is not mitigated. Once decided, this is known as the 'risk appetite' of the organisation. It is defined in terms of the severity of residual risk that can be tolerated. There is, therefore, a very close relationship between the system for scoring risk and the criteria for defining the risk appetite.

Having defined its risk appetite, an organisation must also establish structures and responsibilities for managing all risks and for escalating to a higher level those that are rated above the agreed risk appetite. This will involve the development and maintenance of a range of risk registers for different areas.

As mentioned in 3.2 above, the audit committee should not be directly involved in the process of risk management. However, as the organisation's risk management system underlies the assurance framework, it does have an impact on the committee's work and it will therefore wish to consider whether the organisation's approach to risk is effective and meaningful. Questions it may wish to ask include:

- Is there a comprehensive risk management strategy?
- Is there a clear process for identifying risk?
- Is the organisation's risk appetite clear and understood?
- Are risks clearly assigned to 'owners'?
- Are risks reviewed regularly to ensure their continuing relevance?

It is important to understand that although an organisation's risk management system and the various risk registers it maintains underpin the assurance framework, they are separate processes. The assurance framework's focus is only on the key strategic risks (i.e. those that could prevent the achievement of strategic objectives) whereas risk registers record all risks with only some 'escalated' to the assurance framework itself – the relationship between the two is explained in the case study that follows:

> **Case Study – a Comprehensive Risk Assurance Process**
>
> This NHS trust has an effective 'top down, bottom up' approach to the identification and stratification of risk. The 'top down' element is the establishment of a 'risk stratification matrix' which enables it to define clearly its risk appetite. The 'bottom up' is the system whereby every employee may enter risks onto the risk register. These entries are moderated and classified consistently in accordance with the corporate risk management policy. If the classification ranks them as high in relation to the governing body's risk appetite, they are escalated to the governing body's assurance framework.
>
> The assurance framework is formulated in a way that allows the governing body to focus on key controls and key sources of assurance relating to all the inherent risks to strategic objectives classified as high. Over each twelve month period the governing body requires an update from the lead executive director on each of the key controls and key sources of assurance. The strength of these assurances is reviewed by the audit committee at least once a year. Sometimes this review involves commissioning internal audit to assess the quality of the assurance.

> In this organisation, a compliance team (which is part of the governance team but is managed by internal audit) ensures that both the key controls and key sources of assurance relating to all strategic risks are verified during each annual cycle.

3.4 Reviewing the Assurance Framework's Format and Development

Assurance frameworks vary across organisations and in some instances can be lengthy documents that are not always well understood. This can prevent the framework's effective use for managing the business and its strategic priorities. In other words, to be of real value to an organisation, the assurance framework must be clear, concise and – above all – tailored to the organisation's needs.

The audit committee can help make sure that this is the case by questioning whether the format of its assurance framework and the way in which it is drawn up and used are 'fit for purpose'. In particular, the audit committee will want to seek an assurance that the planning processes underlying the development of the assurance framework and its subsequent maintenance and updating (for example, to reflect changes in understanding of the risk profile and any improvement plans) are sound and that assurances received are acted upon by management. In some organisations, audit committees achieve this by commissioning an annual review of the assurance framework from internal audit.

The Committee may also want to think about how the framework could develop and improve.

> **Assurance Framework Review and Development – Questions for the Audit Committee to Consider**
> - Are we clear about what the assurance framework is for and how it should be used?
> - How do we currently use our assurance framework?
> - How would we like to use it?
> - Who else/what other groups do we think could use it?
> - What do we think about our assurance framework? For example:
>   - Does it do what it's supposed to?
>   - Is its format easy to follow and clear?
>   - What areas do we think need changing, if any?
>   - How would we change them?
> - What is the process for adding new items to the framework?
> - Are all areas covered, including third party assurance?
> - How much comfort does it give us in relation to the running of the organisation?
> - What else gives us comfort and how can we capture those things on the assurance framework?
> - How does it link to the risk register?

3.5 Reviewing the Strategic Objectives in the Assurance Framework

The assurance framework should follow the structure of the organisation's strategic objectives (and associated risks) – as we've seen, these are the high level objectives that are agreed by the governing body that relate to the organisation's overall direction and 'mission'. They should not be confused with operational objectives (and risks) which (although important) relate to an organisation's day-to-day functioning, smooth running and effectiveness – these operational issues should not feature in the assurance framework.

> **The Difference Between Strategic and Operational Risks**
>
> **Strategic risks** relate to the delivery of the organisation's strategic objectives. They have the highest potential for external impact – for example, an adverse effect on engagement with the wider health and social care community and with external stakeholders. Examples include risks to services from competitor organisations; technological or societal change and changing patient demographics.
>
> **Operational risks** relate to the organisation's on-going day-to-day business delivery – for example, patient safety; staff safety; security; information; finance and litigation. Whilst they may have some external impact, operational risks mostly affect internal functioning and services. Depending on the level of risk involved, operational risks are managed at directorate or committee level.
>
> Significant operational risks, which are not effectively managed, can have an impact on the delivery of strategic objectives and organisations therefore need to have a process in place to escalate risk, as required.

In relation to the objectives in an assurance framework, the audit committee's role is to review whether or not they reflect the governing body's priorities and assess the process followed in their compilation.

> **Case Study – Review of the Strategic Objectives**
>
> This audit committee holds a workshop to review the initial assurance framework for the year, following the governing body's approval of the corporate strategic objectives. About six months later, a mid-year review takes place to help ensure that any new risks arising (along with the related assurances linked to the control of those risks) have been included in the assurance framework when appropriate.

3.6 Assessing the Controls in the Assurance Framework

The controls that are set out in the framework to manage the strategic risks are what the organisation relies on from day to day. In assessing these, the audit committee may wish to question whether:

- The controls described are relevant to the risk
- The risks they cover relate to the organisation's strategic objectives
- The controls are complete in terms of adequately covering all of the key risks.

The committee should then seek assurances from management, auditors and any other external sources of assurance as to whether the controls are sound in terms of their design and operation and that they are applied consistently over time.

3.7 Reviewing the Assurances in the Assurance Framework

The assurances in the framework relate to each of the controls and are the key element that enables the governing body to identify those areas that are being well managed and those that may be a cause for concern. The audit committee's role is to consider the overall 'audit needs' of the organisation in terms of these sources of assurance and ensure that there is a plan for them to be received and considered. This should form a key part of the committee's own planning process and requires a thorough review of existing and planned sources of assurance. The results of this review can be looked at during the year using the assurance framework and knowledge of governing body priorities to 're-confirm' the audit plans, particularly in relation to internal audit.

When looking at assurances, it may be helpful for the committee to refer to the 'three lines of defence' conceptual model set out in the Treasury's *Audit and Risk Assurance Committee Handbook*. This splits assurances across three broad categories:

- First line: management assurance from 'front line' or business operational areas
- Second line: oversight of management activity, separate from those responsible for delivery, but not independent of the organisation's management chain
- Third line: independent and more objective assurance, including the role of internal audit and from external bodies.

As well as looking at the sources of assurance, the committee will want to recognise that assurances can be negative or positive:[1]

- Negative: evidence that controls are not working as intended and risks remain unmitigated
- Positive: confirmation that risks are mitigated by the controls with firm evidence to show that the organisation is reasonably managing its risks and that strategic objectives are being delivered.

There are also likely to be other potential sources of assurance where the organisation may be able to gain evidence that the controls on which it is placing reliance are effective.

The assurances themselves take a number of forms (for example, outcome data, process data or reports from inspections or reviews carried out) and are derived from internal or external sources.

---

[1] Please note that the terminology used for assurances (and the underlying meaning) may vary – for example, external auditors may refer to evidence that controls are not working as intended as being a positive assurance as they have found evidence to this effect. The term negative assurance may be used when the auditors have found no evidence that prevents them from concluding that a control is working – but this is not the same as providing an assurance that the control in question is working as it should.

Examples of Sources of Assurance

Internal sources	External sources
Internal audit	External audit
Key performance indicators	Care Quality Commission
Performance reports	Royal College visits
Sub-committee reports	Health Education England
Compliance audit reports	External benchmarking and statistics
Local counter fraud work	Accreditation schemes
Clinical audit	National and regional audits
Staff satisfaction surveys	Peer reviews
Staff appraisals	Feedback from service users
Training records	Local networks (for example, cancer networks)
Training evaluation reports	
Results of internal investigations	Investors in People and other team development tools
Serious untoward incident reports	Feedback from healthcare and third sector partners
Complaints records	
Infection control reports	
Information governance toolkit self-assessment	
Patient advice and liaison services reports	
Workforce and organisational development	
Patient experience surveys and reports	
Internal benchmarking	

Assurances can also be designed specifically for the purpose of providing assurance (for example, a topic in an internal audit plan) or be commissioned for a wider or different purpose (for example, an external inspection).

> **Case Study – Reviewing the Assurances**
>
> This audit committee's annual schedule of work ensures that at least two of the organisation's strategic objectives, as included in the assurance framework, are on the agenda for each meeting. The executive director responsible for that objective is asked to provide the evidence recorded in the 'assurance' column of the assurance framework to members in advance of the meeting. The executive director is also required to attend the next meeting and present a one page paper on the assurance available. The committee members review the information provided and ask questions to assess the adequacy and completeness of the assurances in relation to that objective.

3.8 Assurance Mapping

It is good practice when designing and maintaining the assurance framework to build an 'assurance map' that identifies the sources of assurance that are available and assesses how well they meet the organisation's needs. This is a useful exercise for the audit committee to carry out at the beginning of every year and involves a consideration of:

- The nature and source of the body providing the assurance – for example, is the source internal or external; independent of management or not? What is the providing body's status and reputation?
- The skills and experience of those providing the assurance
- The nature and extent of the work that lies behind the assurance – for example, what approach was taken? Was the organisation visited? Is it a brief overview or an in-depth study? Has comparative data been used?
- How current the assurance is – for example, was it received recently? Is the work on which it is based recent?
- What was the purpose of the review?

For the assurance framework to be effective, it is helpful if internal sources of assurance such as internal audit and clinical audit are involved in the assurance mapping process. This will help ensure that:

- All assurance needs are addressed
- Internal assurance providers remain focused on the organisation's key objectives and priorities
- Best use is made of the available resources.

3.9 Underlying Data

Another key role for the audit committee is to consider whether it has appropriate assurances that the data (including both that which it receives directly and that used to provide assurances on activities and service provision) has undergone quality checks to ensure that it is robust. This involves the committee in looking beyond the messages it receives to critically reviewing the underlying data and assessing whether or not the sources are reliable. This can be particularly challenging in relation to non-financial performance reporting. It is also important to bear in mind that even when another committee or organisation has day-to day responsibility for a particular risk area, the audit committee is ultimately responsible for confirming that it is being managed effectively and that any gaps in assurance are picked up and addressed.

> **Data Quality – Questions for the Committee to Consider**
>
> Is the data source:
>
> - **Valid**: what sources were used – if internal how do we know that the assurance can be relied upon? If external, how was it validated and by whom?
> - **Complete**: did the data collection include all relevant elements and factors?
> - **Up to date**: what period does the data relate to? How recently was it collected?

- **Consistent**: are the messages the committee receives about risks and associated assurances consistent with those that are received and/or monitored by:
  - other committees (for example, a quality committee)
  - service providers (for example, commissioning support units or shared service providers)
  - staff and users of the organisation (for example, governing body members 'walking the floor' and talking directly to NHS staff).
- **Trusted**: how is data viewed within the organisation? Is it believed and used by staff as the basis for action? Or do staff mistrust the data and consider it to be of such poor quality that it does not reflect the activity/service provided and that any problems identified are with the data rather than with the activity?

3.10 Reviewing the Results of Assurances

Having satisfied itself as to the quality of assurances received, the audit committee should review the results of these assurances (either in the round or in relation to a specific risk or objective) and the implications that these have for the achievement of objectives. In doing so, the committee should concentrate on whether:

- The overall objective is being met
- The main controls are operating as expected
- Agreed actions for improvement are being implemented.

The committee will also wish to seek practical evidence that the assurance framework is operating effectively in the organisation. For example, are issues identified in the annual governance statement picked up and acted on in the following year? Is there a link between the organisation's risk register and the performance management system?

3.11 The Assurance Framework and Financial Control

Ensuring that there is effective public accountability, through financial reporting and the maintenance of effective systems of internal financial control remains a key element of the audit committee's work with the review of the annual report and accounts prior to their submission to the governing body being of particular importance. However, financial reporting goes beyond this to cover actual and forecast revenue and capital income and expenditure, and cash flow. The committee should also review the organisation's medium term financial plan and ensure that it is sound and well maintained.

In the context of the assurance framework, the audit committee's role is to ensure that it is reviewing regularly risks and controls relating to financial management and control and assuring itself that the approach is meeting the organisation's statutory duties and business/operational needs. In particular, the committee should review and assess the robustness of management accounts that monitor the financial situation and governing body reports on the organisation's finances. This will involve the committee in considering the integrity, completeness and clarity of financial reporting, taking into consideration the views of external and internal auditors and considering issues of materiality, judgement and estimates that could have a bearing on the accounts. Should concerns arise, the committee should bring these to the attention of the governing body.

> **Case Study – Impact of Materiality**
>
> An unqualified opinion on the accounts from the external auditor gives an assurance that the statements are free from 'material' misstatement. At a large organisation, the threshold for materiality could be £5 million (or more). The audit committee needs to be aware of this and understand that a clean opinion does not necessarily mean that all the figures are correct, just that, based on the testing undertaken by the auditor, the audited financial statements do not contain errors in excess of £5 million (either singly or in aggregate).

In some organisations there will be a finance committee with day-to-day responsibility for financial matters. In such instances, the finance committee will provide assurances to the audit committee with the audit committee retaining ultimately responsible for confirming that the assurances are reliable and that any gaps are picked up and addressed.

Although the Chief Finance Officer (CFO) does not have the same reporting relationship to the audit committee as the respective sets of auditors, he or she is critical to the successful operation of the committee. This is because the CFO has operational responsibility for establishing and maintaining a sound system of internal financial control;[2] is responsible for the production of the annual accounts; is the key contact for the external auditors and is increasingly taking on wider risk management responsibilities. In many organisations, the CFO will also be the key contact at an operational level for internal audit. Consequently, the CFO is a key executive contact with the committee and its Chair and it will be the CFO that the committee will turn to for explanations, clarification and support in relation to financial matters. The committee can also offer the CFO a high profile forum of support when potentially difficult financial control decisions are required.

3.12 The Assurance Framework and Clinical Governance

As the core business of every NHS organisation is healthcare, the audit committee must spend time reviewing healthcare aspects. In particular, it falls to the audit committee to consider the clinical objectives and risks in the assurance framework and to report to the governing body on the related controls and assurances. In this area, provider organisations will be concerned with the clinical care provided within their organisations whereas commissioners will need to take account of the arrangements made by their providers and the extent to which they can obtain assurances about their effectiveness.

There may be a perceived concern about duplication with the audit committee looking at such matters but its role in relation to clinical services is clearly distinguishable. Its objective, at all times, is to satisfy itself that the same level of scrutiny and independent audit in relation to

---

[2] The Accountable/Accounting Officer has statutory responsibility for an organisation's governance, risk management and control framework but will delegate operational responsibility to other directors.

controls and assurances is applied to the risks to **all** strategic objectives, be they clinical, financial or operational. As with financial and operational objectives, the assurance framework is the foundation for the audit committee's work in addressing risks to clinical objectives and satisfying itself that controls are adequate and assurances are sound and sufficient.

Just as the CFO is the main contact for the committee to turn to when looking at financial matters, the audit committee will seek explanations, clarification and support on clinical matters from the relevant director (for example, the Chief Medical Officer or Medical Director) and/or governing body members who will attend committee meetings for this purpose.

3.13 Clinical Risks Arising from Financial Pressures

Financial pressures, when they arise, may lead to changes in clinical services. Both the pressures themselves, and the changes that follow, create the potential for increased risk to the organisation's operations and clinical services that may need to be reflected in the assurance framework. It is for management to identify and mitigate such risks but there is a role for the audit committee to play in recognising the increased risk and satisfying itself that adequate controls are in place and reliable assurances are reported. As we saw in section 1.2, if an organisation fails to assess and deal with these risks effectively, lapses in governance are the likely outcome.

3.14 What Other Assurances Should be Sought?

It is important that the audit committee thinks about what assurances it needs to fulfil its role rather than simply accepting what it is given and assuming that they are sufficient. A good assurance mapping process as described in 3.8 will help ensure that this is the case. Committee members also need to be able to interpret the material they receive and understand its value. The senior member of staff responsible for the committee (the organisation's secretary or governance lead) should advise the audit committee Chair of relevant reports and recommendations that are issued along with an indication of when and how they will be brought to the committee.

For all assurances it is essential that committee members are aware that receiving or noting them is not enough – they must understand the basis on which they have been prepared (including the quality of the underlying data) and the extent of assurance or otherwise which the committee may take from them. This means committee members must be prepared to review assurances critically and use them pro-actively.

Case Study – Quality of Assurances

A number of recent events in the private, financial and public healthcare sectors have demonstrated that senior teams/governing bodies can be blinded by the quantity of evidence and fail to see that it lacks quality and relevance.

Many NHS organisations suffer from having huge volumes of data giving a false sense of assurance. Instead they should be assessing the quality of the evidence based on a number of dimensions – for example:

- The relevance to the item for which it provides assurance
- The opinion on the evidence provided – for example, is it positive, negative or neutral?
- Whether or not it is an internal or external source – for example, from the clinical audit team or the Care Quality Commission
- Whether the assurance is timely or out of date.

Chapter 4: The Work of an Audit Committee

> This chapter focuses on what committee members can expect to do in relation to reviewing the annual accounts and corporate disclosure statements and also looks at how the committee reports on its activities to the governing body.

4.1 How Does the Committee Work in Practice?

The committee conducts most of its business through its regular meetings. However, the Chair will do a certain amount of work outside the committee's meetings (see section 2.8), much of which is in preparation for the meetings.

In terms of specific activities that fall within the committee's remit, members should bear in mind that they must look not just at the reports or statements that they receive but also consider critically the reliability, accuracy and quality of the data upon which these reports are based. They should also consider consistency between reports or statements and be prepared to scrutinise and challenge at all times.

4.2 How Does the Committee Review the Annual Report and Accounts?

The committee is required to review the annual report and accounts before they are submitted to the governing body for formal adoption. Usually this involves considering a report from the Chief Finance Officer (CFO) in April or May. The ISA 260 report to those charged with governance[1] from the external auditor should also be received by the audit committee at this stage (see section 5.4.6).

The audit committee's review of the accounts is an important step in the governing body's approval process and provides an opportunity for constructive challenge and scrutiny of the organisation's financial information and systems of control. Accordingly committee members need to be able to understand the annual report and accounts before recommending their approval.

When reviewing the accounts the Committee may wish to pay particular attention to the following aspects:

- Compliance with relevant requirements
- Changes in accounting policies
- Changes in accounting practice due to changes in accounting standards
- Changes in estimation techniques
- Significant judgements made in preparing the financial statements
- Significant adjustments resulting from the audit
- Any un-adjusted mis-statements in the financial statements
- Explanations for significant variances
- Any letters of representation.

---

[1] *International Standard on Auditing (UK and Ireland) 260 – Communication with those Charged with Governance.*

Case Studies – Reviewing the Annual Accounts

Case study 1

The presentation of the audited accounts to the audit committee at this organisation was accompanied by a briefing that outlined:

- Performance against all financial targets
- Reasons behind the big moves between financial years
- Changes in, and compliance with, accounting policies and practices
- Major areas of judgement
- Significant adjustments arising from the audit
- The sources of assurance available to the audit committee to help it support the recommendation to the governing body to adopt the accounts.

This was followed by a lengthy and informed discussion on a range of issues by the non-executive directors.

Case study 2

This organisation arranged an informal meeting of the audit committee, one week prior to its formal meeting, where the CFO presented the full financial statements. The external audit manager also attended to provide details of audit findings and what these meant for the accounts approval process. Time invested in the informal meeting enabled a more productive formal audit committee meeting as the questions asked were more informed and relevant indicating that the NEDs understood the financial statements and the accounts and audit process.

4.3 How Does the Committee Review the Annual Governance Statement?

All NHS organisations produce an annual governance statement that forms part of the annual report and accounts. This statement focuses on the stewardship of the organisation and draws together position statements and evidence on governance, risk management and control, to provide a coherent and consistent reporting mechanism. Although there is no prescribed format the statement must cover a number of areas including:

- Scope of the organisation's Accounting/Accountable Officer's responsibilities
- Information about the organisation's governance framework
- A description of how risk is assessed and managed
- Information about how the risk and control framework works
- A review of the effectiveness of risk management and internal control
- Any significant control issues and how they are being addressed.

Each year, guidance is issued to NHS organisations about the preparation of the annual governance statement. There is also a useful explanation of what these statements are designed to achieve in Annex 3.1 of the Treasury's publication *Managing Public Money*.[2]

---

[2] *Managing Public Money*, HM Treasury, 2013:
https://www.gov.uk/government/publications/managing-public-money

The audit committee is required to review the draft statement before it is submitted to the governing body for its scrutiny. To ensure that deadlines are met, this usually involves considering a report from the Accounting/Accountable Officer before the end of May. Issues that the committee may wish to consider are:

- Whether the statement includes all the elements required in relevant guidance
- Whether there are any inconsistencies between the statements made and reports the committee has received from auditors or other sources of assurance
- Whether any significant control issues or gaps in control or assurance recorded in the statement are consistent with reports the committee has received
- Whether the statement gives a balanced view of the organisation's governance arrangements over the last year.

The committee is also likely to consider the annual Head of Internal Audit Opinion at this meeting as it is designed to be one of the elements that informs the annual governance statement.

The committee will then report to the governing body confirming that the draft governance statement is consistent with the view of the committee on the organisation's system of internal control and that it supports the governing body's approval of the statement, subject to any reasonable limitations that the committee may draw attention to.

To be able to carry out this review effectively, the audit committee will wish to look out for any possible problem areas or gaps throughout the year and discuss them as and when they arise.

4.4 How Does the Committee Review Evidence Relating to the Organisation's Continuing 'Fitness to Function'?

The Committee will wish to review the processes by which evidence is produced to show that the organisation is fulfilling regulatory requirements relating to its existence as a functioning business. For example:

- Fitness to remain registered with the Care Quality Commission
- Compliance with terms of authorisation for CCGs
- Compliance with the terms and requirements of Monitor's licence
- Compliance with the sustainability guidance outlined in the NHS Trust Development Authority's planning guidance[3] and *Accountability Framework*.[4]

In each case, the committee will look at the rigour of the process for compiling the evidence and the quality and reliability of the underlying data upon which it is based. This will involve linking with other committees that play a role and confirming that the assurances they provide

---

[3] *Securing Sustainability – Planning Guidance for NHS Trust Boards 2014/2015 – 2018/19*, NHS TDA, 2013: www.ntda.nhs.uk/blog/2013/12/23/planning-guidance/

[4] *Delivering High Quality Care for Patients: The Accountability Framework*, NHS TDA, 2013: www.ntda.nhs.uk/blog/2013/05/03/delivering-high-quality-care-for-patients-the-accountabilty-framework-2/

are reliable and that any gaps are picked up and addressed. The audit committee will also wish to review all statements made and assurances given to ensure that they are consistent with the committee's own knowledge and assurances.

4.5 How Does the Committee Review the Quality Accounts?

All providers of acute care (including mental health, ambulance and disability learning trusts) are required to produce an annual quality account (also referred to as a quality report) in line with the statutory requirement set out in the *Health Act 2009*. The aim is to 'enhance accountability to the public and engage the leaders of an organisation in their quality improvement agenda' by reporting the continuous improvement in the quality of the services provided. A core set of quality indicators must be included in all NHS bodies' quality accounts as prescribed in statutory instruments supporting the 2009 Act and guidance issued by the Department of Health.[5] Each affected organisation's chief executive[6] is required to sign a statement of accountability for the quality account covering two elements:

- Whether the data reported in the quality account is reported accurately – this is not only about the reliability of the data but also about its interpretation
- Whether the quality account is representative in its reporting of the services provided and the issues of concern to its stakeholders.

Parts of the quality accounts are also reviewed by auditors as set down in guidance issued by Monitor and (until 2013/14) the Audit Commission.[7]

The audit committee's role is to consider the rigour of the processes for identifying and defining the services to be reported and the improvements planned as well as the processes for compiling and interpreting the data used as indicators of performance. The committee then reports to the full governing body on the robustness of the processes behind the quality accounts.

4.6 How Should the Committee Report During the Year?

The audit committee's work should be aligned to the governing body's agenda and as a result, its in-year reporting to the governing body is of great significance. Specifically, the committee alerts the governing body to the results of its reviews of assurances as well as any 'exceptional' issues that arise during the year and which fall within its area of interest. In addition, the governing body expects to receive reports arising from the committee's review of the annual report and accounts and statutory declarations as well as any other matters requested by the governing body at the start of the year. Normally, reports from the audit committee should

---

[5] Information about quality accounts (including links to regulations and guidance): www.nhs.uk/aboutNHSChoices/professionals/healthandcareprofessionals/quality-accounts/Pages/about-quality-accounts.aspx

[6] The phrase used in the 2010 regulations is 'the most senior employee for a body corporate'.

[7] All NHS foundation trusts are reviewed. However, from 2014/15, the Audit Commission is not specifying requirements for the external assurance of quality accounts. Alternative arrangements will be put in place in due course.

take the form of clear concise minutes, presented by the audit committee Chair with an oral report or written summary highlighting the key messages – for example, new risks, new assurances and progress with actions to close gaps in control or assurance.

4.7 How Should the Committee Report at Year End?

In line with best practice in other sectors, the audit committee should prepare an annual report to the full governing body that sets out how the committee has discharged its responsibilities and met its terms of reference.[8]

The report should summarise the committee's work during the year and (as a minimum) confirm that:

- The organisation's system of risk management is adequate in identifying risks and allowing the governing body to understand the appropriate management of those risks
- The committee has reviewed and used the assurance framework and believes that it is fit for purpose and that the 'comprehensiveness' of the assurances and the reliability and integrity of the sources of assurance are sufficient to support the governing body's decisions and declarations
- There are no outstanding areas of significant duplication or omission in the organisation's systems of governance that have come to the committee's attention.

In addition, the report should highlight the main areas that the committee has reviewed and any particular concerns or issues that it has addressed. These could include:

- The reliability and quality of the organisation's financial reporting systems that 'sit' behind the financial position reported to the governing body
- Any significant issues that the committee has considered in relation to the financial statements
- Any major break-down in internal control that has led to a significant loss in one form or another
- Any major weakness in the governance systems that has exposed, or continues to expose, the organisation to an unacceptable risk
- The reliability and quality of clinical information systems and clinical auditing processes and the extent to which the governing body can take assurance from these
- An assessment of the performance of the external auditor
- The value of any non-audit services provided by the external auditors.

The committee's annual report is presented to the governing body promptly after the financial year-end but before it considers the organisation's annual report and statutory declarations. As a result, the committee's annual report will make a general reference to its role in these matters but its detailed opinions will be the subject of subsequent, separate reports to the governing body.

---

[8] For FTs the requirement to report to the Council of Governors and the information that should be included is set out in section C.3 of Monitor's *Code of Governance*.

Best Practice – the Audit Committee's Annual Report

- The report should not be long (3 or 4 pages should be sufficient) and may be drafted by the committee's secretary under the direction of the committee's Chair
- The committee Chair should take overall responsibility for the report's preparation and share drafts of the report with committee members
- The final draft report should be shared with the internal and external auditors, to ensure that it is consistent with their understanding, and with any other regular attendees to the committee, such as the CFO. However, the report must be owned by the committee itself
- The report should go to all members of the governing body in advance of the meeting to agree the annual report and accounts
- If the report includes any significant issues, these should be discussed by the audit committee Chair with the Chair of the governing body prior to the report being presented to the full governing body
- Rather than just focus on process and the number/type of assurances considered during the year, the report should seek to identify the outcome of the committee's work, its conclusions and actions taken.

Chapter 5: Working with Other Committees and Auditors

> In fulfilling the roles described in previous chapters, the audit committee will want to rely on the organisation's internal arrangements and auditors. This chapter describes its relationship with other committees; with internal, external and clinical auditors and with those involved in counter (or anti-) fraud and security activities. In particular it looks at the assurances the audit committee can expect to receive from each and suggests how it can assess their value and reliability. There are also references to governance between organisations (an area of increasing importance with the expansion of shared services and partnership working) and whistle blowing.

5.1 How Should the Audit Committee Relate to Other Committees?

The audit committee will need to have an effective relationship with other key committees that may exist within an organisation (for example, finance, quality, risk management, governance and remuneration) so that it can understand what the linkages are and what each covers. To be able to do this, every organisation should have a 'map' setting out how committees fit together and what their responsibilities are. This should distinguish between formal committees of the governing body and informal groups that are often set up for a specific task and finish purpose.

It is extremely important that the roles of other committees are not merged with those of the audit committee, as this would impair the independence the latter needs to be able to review and comment on:

- The information and assurances provided by these other committees – for example, are their reports accurate and based on sound evidence?
- The overall effectiveness of the arrangements in place to ensure high quality, effective governance and risk management.

To ensure that this is the case, the respective terms of reference for each committee should make clear their roles with no duplication or inconsistencies. For example, where there is a risk committee, the audit committee's role is not to duplicate what it does but rather to ensure (on behalf of the governing body) that the overall system for risk management is in place and effective. Operational responsibility for the management of risk lies with the risk committee and senior managers.

Similarly, if the Chair of the audit committee chairs other committees (as could be the case in a CCG), it is essential that effective safeguards are in place to ensure that the audit committee's independence is not compromised.

> **Case Study – Relationship with Other Key Committees**
>
> This audit committee Chair invites the Chair of the risk committee to sit in at audit committee meetings at least once a year to explore their respective roles and to assess the effectiveness of the relationship between the committees. A similar invitation is extended to the Chairs of other key committees (for example, clinical governance and quality) from time to time.

5.2 How do the Auditors Support the Audit Committee's Work?

Although, the committee's name refers to 'audit', this does not alter the fact that the majority of assurances to the committee come from management. In addition, the committee will quite rightly look to auditors (internal, external and clinical) to provide a critical element of independent assurance.

It is not the role of the audit committee to manage the organisation's audit functions; rather it should use the internal, external and clinical auditors to assist it in meeting its needs, along with other sources of advice and assurance. This means that the audit committee should actively review the plans of the auditors and understand the distinct and separate roles that each plays.

Before we move on to look in detail at how the audit committee works with each set of auditors, it is helpful to understand their nature.

5.2.1 Who are the internal auditors?

Internal auditors may be employed directly by an organisation; bought in on a shared service basis; provided through an NHS consortium, or contracted in from a commercial firm. In all cases, the audit committee will want to assess the quality of the service and the extent to which it meets the organisation's needs. If a new appointment is under consideration, the audit committee will expect to be consulted and involved in the process.

In contrast to external audit where the role is closely defined, there is scope for the audit committee to influence the internal audit strategy and request work that focuses on its own assurance needs (and thereby the needs of the governing body).

5.2.2 Who are the external auditors?

At present, external auditors are appointed by the Audit Commission for CCGs and non-foundation NHS trusts and by an FT's Council of Governors in NHS foundation trusts. The role of external auditors is set out in the Audit Commission's *Code of Audit Practice* or Monitor's *Audit Code for NHS Foundation Trusts*. As a result, there is less opportunity for the audit committee to have an impact on what they do.

In the case of FTs, the audit committee supports the Council of Governors by providing it with the information it needs to set criteria for appointing, re-appointing and removing the external auditors – for example about external auditors' performance. The Council of Governors takes the lead in agreeing these criteria with the audit committee. Although audit committees in other NHS bodies have no formal role in the appointment of external auditors, they will also wish to monitor the quality of their work.

After the Audit Commission is abolished in 2015 and once existing contracts with external auditors expire, the regime for appointing external auditors will change with all NHS bodies appointing their own auditors as set out in the *Local Audit and Accountability Act 2014*. In practice this means that external auditors will begin to be appointed under the new regime from 2017 (although some contracts may run until 2020 if the government decides to extend them).

Following the Audit Commission's closure, the National Audit Office will issue the *Audit Code of Practice* and it will then apply to all NHS organisations, including FTs.

5.2.3 Who are the clinical auditors?

The focus of clinical auditors is on driving improvement in clinical practice. This means that their relationship with the audit committee is more akin to that of, say, a risk committee, with the audit committee's focus on ensuring (on behalf of the governing body) that the overall arrangements for clinical audit are effective. As with internal audit, there is some scope for the audit committee to influence the clinical audit strategy.

5.3 How Does Internal Audit Support the Audit Committee's Work?

5.3.1 What does internal audit do?

An effective audit committee is dependent, in many respects, on the existence of an effective internal audit function as it is a key part of the organisation's internal control environment. It is therefore important that the audit committee understands what internal audit involves. The *Public Sector Internal Audit Standards*[1] that apply to all non-foundation NHS trusts and CCGs[2] describe internal audit as 'an independent, objective assurance and consulting activity designed to add value and improve an organisation's operations'. This means that its role embraces two key areas:

1. The provision of an independent and objective opinion to the Accountable/Accounting Officer, the governing body, and the audit committee on the degree to which risk management, control and governance support the achievement of the organisation's agreed objectives
2. The provision of an independent and objective consultancy service specifically to help line management improve the organisation's risk management, control and governance arrangements.

The audit committee will find the *Public Sector Internal Audit Standards* an essential source of reference for understanding what they can expect from internal audit and assessing the service provided. These standards require the 'purpose, authority and responsibility' of internal audit to be 'formally defined in an internal audit charter, consistent with the Definition of Internal Audit, the Code of Ethics and the Standards'.

The cycle of approving internal audit plans and monitoring progress reports, culminating in the annual Head of Internal Audit Opinion on the system of internal control, are a key feature of the audit committee's work and internal auditors should attend every audit committee meeting for this reason. The audit committee will also wish to direct internal audit to look at

---

[1] *Public Sector Internal Audit Standards*, 2013:
https://www.gov.uk/government/publications/public-sector-internal-audit-standards
[2] Although these standards are not mandatory for FTs, Monitor bought them to FTs' attention in its December 2012 monthly bulletin.

particular areas of concern during the year and internal audit providers should be flexible enough to react to any such requests.

The value of internal audit to the audit committee derives from the 'risk based approach' to internal audit that professional standards require. The benefits manifest themselves in two key areas:

- Internal audit opinions – these are not limited to the extent of compliance with known controls but report on the relevance of the controls themselves in relation to the risks to the organisation
- Internal audit plans – the plans are based on a risk assessment of all activities in the organisation (clinical, financial and other), using the organisation's objectives and risks as recorded in the assurance framework as a primary source. This means that both multi-year and annual audit plans are developed to reflect the fact that not every topic warrants an annual review.

> **Internal Audit Objectives – Best Practice and Questions to Consider**
>
> - Is there a written statement defining internal audit's objectives, responsibilities, authority and reporting lines (often referred to as an 'internal audit charter')? Does the committee see and review this?
> - Does the charter comply with the *Public Sector Internal Audit Standards* and set out the scope of internal audit activities; internal audit's position within the organisation; its authority to access records, personnel and physical properties relevant to the performance of audit assignments/reviews and a set of performance indicators that monitor the overall quality of the service?

5.3.2 The status of internal audit

It is important that the Head of Internal Audit has a right of access to the Chair of the audit committee at any time, and it should be clear that management cannot restrict or censor this access. For FTs, Monitor's *Code of Governance* (paragraph C.2.d) states that if an FT has an internal audit service its head 'should have a direct reporting line to the board or to the audit committee to bring the requisite degree of independence and objectivity to the role.'

It is good practice for the audit committee's Chair to meet informally with the Head of Internal Audit from time to time, perhaps in advance of each audit committee meeting.

> **Internal Audit Status: Best Practice and Questions to Consider**
>
> - Does the Head of Internal Audit have direct access to the audit committee and governing body?
> - Are any scope restrictions placed on internal audit and, if so, who establishes them?
> - Does internal audit report directly to an appropriate level of management that will ensure that audit findings are given due weight and attention?
> - Are the internal auditors free from any operational responsibilities that could impair their objectivity?

5.3.3 How should the committee review the internal audit plan?

Internal audit submits a planning document to the audit committee for approval prior to the start of each financial year.[3] Although there is no set format for this document, it should:

- Describe how the internal audit plan has been developed (including details of who has been involved and evidence that there is 'buy in' across the organisation)
- Satisfy the committee that it is risk based and linked to the assurance framework
- Show that internal audit has worked with management to ensure that the assurances needed by the committee (and governing body) are addressed and that it is sufficiently well balanced across all that the organisation does
- Give enough information so that the committee can understand whether the work planned is of sufficient breadth and depth
- Indicate how internal audit intends to co-ordinate its work with other internal assurance providers to ensure the best use of resources
- Indicate how internal audit intends to work with external bodies that carry out work for the organisation
- Show that internal audit has understood and allowed for the expectations of external auditors.

The audit committee may wish to participate in this planning process – for example, by convening an annual planning meeting. In some organisations, members of the quality committee may also attend to ensure close coordination – this can be particularly helpful when internal audit also provides assurance to the quality committee.

At a more detailed level, the annual internal audit plan should include information about the purposes, scope and level of priority of each assignment. This will include:

- The approach that will be taken for each assignment – for example, whether it will be a high level review or detailed testing
- Any new areas that will be covered and why
- Reasons for any areas not covered in the plan – for example, if assurances come from elsewhere
- The resources needed in terms of time and skills
- Linkages between the planned activities and the assurance framework.

The plan should also include an allowance (i.e. in terms of resources) for maintaining a sound understanding of organisational risks throughout the year to ensure that changing circumstances and emerging risks are spotted and addressed. There may also be a need on occasion to address urgent issues that arise in year – for example, to extend an audit if initial findings indicate a concern. The audit committee (and management) should approve any changes to the plan that result.

---

[3] On occasion, other planning processes may be delayed and as result it may not be possible to reflect fully all organisational risks before the financial year starts. In such circumstances audit committees may decide to approve a draft internal audit plan with a further 'sign off' process taking place once all planning processes have been finalised.

Given that the audit committee has a key responsibility to review internal control and risk management systems and that internal audit is a primary source of assurance in this respect, it is essential that when approving the plan, the audit committee is confident that the work it describes will be sufficient for its purposes and that internal audit has enough resources to deliver it. To help the committee make this assessment, it will wish to have available at the relevant meeting both the assurance map (to show how internal audit fits into the wider process) and the assurance framework. The Accountable/Accounting Officer should also be in attendance as the work that internal audit does is a key element in the production of the annual governance statement that he or she must sign.

> **Case Study – Internal Audit Plan**
>
> In many organisations, the audit committee also considers projects that have been proposed by internal audit but 'stood down' or deferred by the executive. For example, management may feel that problems in a particular area are well understood and any internal audit work is therefore unnecessary – perhaps because remedial action is already underway or there is an action plan in place. The audit committee can either accept that these risks are being mitigated or ask internal audit to reinstate the project – this may happen when the committee feels that either the risks themselves or plans for improvement are not sufficiently well defined.
>
> Similarly, in circumstances where systems are being extensively redesigned, internal audit may have an input to the design process and advising on governance, risk and control considerations. The audit committee may wish to assess whether internal audit has identified such initiatives and engaged appropriately.

It is not possible to publish a model internal audit plan as each one is designed to reflect the local risks and available/required sources of assurance within a particular organisation. However, being aware of some of the key high level issues that should be covered will help an audit committee with its review and assessment.

> **Key Issues that an Internal Audit Plan Should Cover**
>
> **1. Audit risk assessment**
> Internal audit should regularly assess the level of maturity of the organisation's risk management system as this affects the design of its own plan. For example, a mature risk management system allows internal audit to use the organisation's own assessment of risk to determine the content of its plan. However, where the risk management system is still being developed or is patchy, internal audit will undertake its own risk assessments, either for parts (or all) of the organisation.
>
> A top down assessment of risk, using the assurance framework and discussions with managers, should be carried out to allow a focus on key priorities. A bottom up risk assessment using a range of sources such as risk registers; sources of assurance (including internal audit's own prior assessments); external inspections; performance reports and other

governing body papers should be undertaken to confirm the completeness and accuracy of top down sources.

2. Core financial systems

The audit committee has a responsibility to monitor the integrity of internal financial control as this is critical to the success of an organisation. Sufficient resources should therefore be invested to provide necessary assurances based on the organisation's risk profile. As the external audit process is likely to rely on the work of internal audit in this area, both sets of auditors should liaise to ensure that their expectations are defined and delivered.

3. Governance

An effectively designed governance framework with high levels of compliance is critical to the success of an organisation. The audit committee has ultimate responsibility for reviewing these arrangements* and the Accountable/Accounting Officer has a responsibility to comment on them in the annual governance statement. Internal audit should invest sufficient resources to provide necessary assurances in this area in relation to its design and application based on the organisation's risk profile.

4. Risk management and the assurance framework

An effectively designed risk management system (including the assurance framework) is critical to the success of an organisation. The audit committee has ultimate responsibility to review these arrangements* and the Accountable/Accounting Officer has a responsibility to comment on their effectiveness in the annual governance statement. Internal audit should invest sufficient resources to provide necessary assurances in this area in relation to its design and application based on the organisation's risk profile.

5. Key systems

A number of systems are key to the success of an organisation – for example, to ensure compliance with legislation and regulations; to deliver services to performance expectations or to support the delivery of business objectives. Examples include the ICT network; the performance management system and CQC standards compliance monitoring systems. Internal audit should invest sufficient resources to provide necessary assurances in this area based on the organisation's risk profile.

6. Consultancy

This is a demand-led element of the internal audit service's activities and while some topics may be identified in an annual plan, part of the value of consultancy lies in having sufficient capacity and flexibility to be able to respond to priorities that emerge during the year.

Consultancy and advisory assignments tend to focus on diagnosing problems and/or designing solutions. They are not undertaken primarily to provide assurance. Internal audit needs to take care when accepting consultancy assignments as its independence must be safeguarded. For example, internal audit should not advise on the design of improvements to a system and then undertake an assurance audit of that system as the objectivity of the findings could be compromised.

* In some organisations a dedicated risk committee or the governing body itself may also have a role.

The relative resources allocated to each of the key areas identified above and the overall resources applied to internal audit are a matter for each Head of Internal Audit to recommend and for each organisation's management and audit committee to take a view on. In making these judgements, it is helpful to bear in mind that:

- The plan is unlikely to be static – topics will move in and out as the assessment of risk and control in each area changes (hopefully for the better). This means that over a period of years assurance on a wider range of topics will be received by the audit committee.
- Not every topic that warrants a review needs to be covered every year. Multi-year plans based on risk can include some topics on a two or three-yearly cycle which means that a greater range of topics can be covered over the cycle.

> **Internal Audit Plans – Best Practice and Questions to Consider**
> - Are there clear protocols that set out the way in which internal audit will relate to and work with other internal assurance functions (clinical audit, quality, risk management etc.) and is there evidence of coordination between these parties concerning the planning of assurances for the assurance framework?
> - Are there clear protocols that set out the way in which internal audit will relate to and work with external organisations that carry out work for the organisation – for example, shared services centres and commissioning support units?
> - Is the audit plan derived from clear processes based on risk assessments and strategic objectives that can be reconciled to the assurance framework and satisfy the committee's assurance needs?
> - Does the plan take into account the risk maturity of the organisation?
> - How is the scope of internal audit work decided? What are the relative emphases given to internal control reviews; policy compliance reviews; value for money audits and consultancy assignments?
> - Is the technical knowledge, skills and experience of internal audit staff sufficient to ensure that duties are performed to an appropriate standard?
> - Is the work of the internal auditors properly planned, completed, supervised and reviewed?
> - Is the internal audit plan prepared following consultation with other assurance providers?
> - Is there appropriate cooperation with external auditors?

To give an idea of the range of work that audit committees can expect internal audit planning to consider in both a provider and commissioning organisation, see appendix D.

5.3.4 How should the committee review internal audit assignment reports?

Having been involved in agreeing (and approving) internal audit's planned coverage for the year, the committee will expect to see regular reports about the results of each assignment. A periodic summary report of audits completed against the plan enables the committee to monitor progress in receiving the assurances anticipated. The committee may wish to see the full report from each assignment as it is completed but in any case will need to know the level of assurance that has been awarded (for example, full, significant, limited or no assurance) and the main recommendations for improvement that have been made to management. In this way the committee will receive prompt notification of the findings and assurances that internal audit has reported.

An important role for the audit committee is to monitor the implementation of agreed audit recommendations and it should ensure that the organisation has in place a robust process that does this. In particular, regular progress reports should be provided to the committee identifying any recommendations that have not been implemented within agreed timescales. Where the audit committee and/or Head of Internal Audit are concerned about the lack of implementation in a particular area, the audit committee can assist by asking the operational manager to attend a meeting and explain.

> **Internal Audit Assignments – Best Practice and Questions to Consider**
> - The audit committee will wish to establish that the report arising from each assignment is issued to management on a timely basis
> - The audit committee will require internal audit to prioritise its findings against defined levels of assurance – this will then clearly indicate the importance of each finding and the degree of urgency attached to each action point
> - The audit committee should ensure that once internal audit has agreed its findings and recommendations with management, the actions required are allocated to named individuals to implement in line with agreed timescales
> - The audit committee should monitor the implementation of agreed actions by a variety of means – the aim being to review whether important recommendations have been actioned by management and that either assurance levels have improved and/or risks reduced. In each case the committee will wish to consider whether to invite the relevant senior manager to report on progress
> - The committee will wish to ensure that if internal audit recommendations to management are not acted upon, there is a process for their escalation.

5.3.5 How should the committee review the Head of Internal Audit's annual opinion?

The Head of Internal Audit is required to give a formal annual opinion to the governing body and Accountable/Accounting Officer via the audit committee on the overall adequacy and effectiveness of the organisation's risk management, control and governance processes. This opinion supports and informs the annual governance statement (see section 4.3) and includes a consideration of:

- The design and operation of the system of assurance and the assurance framework
- The findings from the range of internal audit assignments completed during the year
- The evidence required to show that the organisation is fulfilling regulatory requirements relating to its existence as a functioning business.

The audit committee will receive an annual report from the Head of Internal Audit expanding on these opinions and informing it about internal audit performance.

Working with Other Committees and Auditors

> **Annual Head of Internal Audit Opinion: Best Practice and Questions to Consider**
> - The audit committee will wish to establish that the scope of the opinion covers all of the key activities planned, including any areas that were requested during the year
> - The audit committee will wish to satisfy itself that the opinion is consistent with the detailed reports received during the preceding year and that it takes account of any post year-end events if necessary
> - The audit committee Chair will want to report the opinion to the governing body as evidence to be used in compiling the annual governance statement.

5.3.6 How should the committee review the effectiveness of internal audit?

Given the importance of internal audit to an audit committee, it is essential that the committee is happy with the quality of service provided. Audit committees should therefore review the function's effectiveness each year, taking into consideration professional and regulatory requirements. External auditors' views may be helpful here as they can give an assessment of its adequacy.

> **The Effectiveness of Internal Audit – Best Practice and Questions to Consider**
> - Are internal auditors asked about their internal systems of quality assurance and quality control, and do they provide feedback on the results of this?
> - Does the audit committee receive periodically (i.e. no less than every five years) an independent external report on the internal audit service provider's adherence to the *Public Sector Internal Audit Standards*?
> - Has the committee sought the views of the external auditors on the adequacy of the internal audit service?

5.3.7 What is the committee's role in relation to third party assurances and hosted bodies and how does internal audit fit in?

It is important that audit committees are clear about the third party assurances that they require and the format that they need to follow – this can be included in the assurance mapping process described in section 3.8.

In practice this means that the audit committee will wish to be aware if a significant activity is shared with (or bought in from) another organisation – for example, shared financial services and commissioning support. It is likely that the organisations providing these services will have their own internal audit arrangements. Audit committees of organisations using the services will therefore expect to receive assurances from those internal auditors to confirm that risks in the services provided to them are adequately managed and mitigated with appropriate controls. Audit committees of organisations providing such services will wish to satisfy themselves that their own internal audit is sufficient to provide:

- Assurance that risks to the host are adequately controlled
- The third party assurances that user organisations require.

One approach that is in widespread use is to require third parties to follow *ISAE 3402: Assurance reports on controls at a service organisation*. An ISAE 3402 report[4] gives stakeholders assurance over the key controls tested within the scope of the work. It is important that bodies relying on these reports understand the scope of the testing commissioned by the service organisation from their auditors, and are satisfied that it appropriately covers all key objectives and risks. Any gaps should be raised with the partner organisation with a view to either seeking alternative assurance or extending the scope of the ISAE 3402 report.

The audit committee will also wish to know if their organisation 'hosts' another organisation that serves the wider NHS. The hosted body will have its own management and committee structure but its budget may be significant to the host organisation. The audit committee will therefore wish to consider whether there is sufficient internal audit coverage in place to provide assurance over any risks to their own organisation that the hosted body might represent. Such assurance might come from the hosted body's own internal audit service but if nothing is in place the audit committee will want to take the initiative in ensuring that appropriate internal audit is established.

The increasing trend for joint and partnership working in the provision of services adds a further dimension to governance between organisations and often involves organisations outside the NHS. In such arrangements, risks tend to arise at the borders between one organisation and another and are exacerbated if the respective roles and responsibilities of the partners are not clearly defined, understood and written down. Again, the audit committee will wish to know about any such arrangements and ensure that appropriate internal audit is established.

5.4 How Does External Audit Support the Audit Committee's Work?

5.4.1 What does external audit do?

The objectives of the external auditors fall under two broad headings – to review and report on:

- The audited body's financial statements (including its annual governance statement and quality account – see chapter 4)
- Whether the audited body has made proper arrangements for securing economy, efficiency and effectiveness in its use of resources.

In each case, the audit committee will expect to see the resulting conclusions.

5.4.2 The status of external audit

External auditors are usually invited to attend every audit committee meeting, and the cycle of approving and monitoring the progress of external audit plans and reports, culminating in the

---

[4] There are two types of ISAE 3402 report – type 1 states whether controls were operating at a point in time; Type 2 is more detailed and looks at the operation of controls over a period of time (for example, part of a year). Audit committees should understand the nature of the report they receive.

opinion on the annual report and accounts, is central to the work of the committee. The appointed external auditor should have a right of access to the Chair of the audit committee at any time.

5.4.3 How should the committee review the external audit strategy and Plan?

The appointed auditor should prepare an audit strategy. The strategy should be developed to deliver an opinion on the annual accounts and a conclusion on proper arrangements, and will take into account the audit needs of the organisation, as assessed by the appointed auditor, using a risk-based approach. The audit committee should agree the strategy.

External audit should also prepare an annual audit plan, designed to implement the audit strategy, for approval by the audit committee. This annual plan should set out details of the work to be carried out, providing sufficient detail for the audit committee and other recipients to understand the purpose and scope of the defined work and the level of priority. The audit committee should discuss with the external auditors the main issues and parameters for audit planning in the meeting before the annual audit plan is due to be approved. This allows committee members time and space to:

- Discuss the organisation's audit needs
- Reflect on the previous year's experience
- Be updated on likely changes and new issues
- Ensure coordination with other bodies and assurance providers.

In reviewing the draft plan committee members should concentrate on the outputs from the plan, and what they will receive from the external auditors, balanced against an understanding of the auditors' statutory functions. Review of the audit fee is also important, with the focus on its appropriateness in the context of the organisation's needs whilst recognising that there are statutory functions that external auditors must carry out.

Once agreed, the annual audit plan should be kept under review and amended to reflect changing priorities and emerging audit needs. The audit committee should approve any material changes to the plan.

External audit should be working with both management and other assurance functions to optimise its level of coverage. The committee will want to see, and gain assurance, that duplication with internal audit is minimised wherever possible, consistent with the requirements of *ISA (UK and Ireland) 610* that external audit should not direct the work of internal audit and must be satisfied as to the role of internal audit as a whole and review and 're-perform' similar items for any piece of work on which it intends to place reliance. In practice this means that external audit will wish to liaise with internal audit so that it understands its activities and how they fit in with its own strategy. Internal audit will also wish to leave a sufficiently detailed 'audit trail' to allow external audit to be able to 're-perform' work when necessary – although this is not likely to occur routinely.

As mentioned in 5.3.6, the audit committee will also find external audit's view on the adequacy of internal audit valuable.

> **External Audit Arrangements – Best Practice and Questions to Consider**
> - The audit committee should expect to see audit plans that are based on a clear assessment of audit risk that takes account of the key strategic risks facing the organisation
> - The audit committee should approve the annual plan and the associated fees, although in so doing it needs to recognise that external auditors have statutory duties to fulfil
> - External auditors need to plan work to discharge their responsibilities but the audit committee should review the work they propose to carry out and seek to ensure that it addresses the key risks and adds value to the organisation. In this latter respect, external audit's work should not replace activity that is part of the management function, or could be achieved by a better use of other resources (for example, by re-allocating management duties or using an internal assurance function)
> - The audit committee should ensure that the external auditors understand the organisation's wider position in the health economy and consider the risks associated with partners/other stakeholders, and the potential impact on the quality of healthcare services
> - External auditors should be asked about their own internal systems of quality assurance and quality control, and be prepared to give the committee feedback
> - The Chair of the audit committee should have good relationships with the lead from external audit (at the Partner/Director level) so that any adverse reports (for example, a Public Interest Report) do not come as a surprise
> - The audit committee will wish to consider whether any scope restrictions are placed on external audit and, if so, who establishes them
> - The audit committee will wish to consider whether the external auditors are free from any conflicts that could impair their objectivity
> - The audit committee will wish to consider whether the technical knowledge and experience of the external audit staff is sufficient to ensure that duties are performed to an appropriate standard.

5.4.4 *How should the committee deal with non-audit services?*

It should be noted that in some circumstances an NHS organisation's external auditors may provide other additional services that are outside the scope of the audit as defined in 5.4.1 – for example, they may provide advice on tax issues. Where this is the case, it is good practice for the audit committee to approve a policy for considering and managing any such services. Monitor's *Code of Governance* (provision C.3.2) requires audit committees in FTs to 'develop and implement policy on the engagement of the external auditor to supply non-audit services, taking into account relevant ethical guidance regarding the provision of non-audit services by the external audit firm.'

If the proportion of non-audit services becomes significant, the audit committee may need to consider whether or not there is a need to change the external auditors.

> **Case Study – Non Audit Services Policy**
>
> In this organisation, the policy includes the following provisions:
>
> - If non-audit work carried out by its external auditor exceeds a pre-set percentage, approval is needed from the audit committee[5]
> - The proportion of audit *versus* non-audit work is reviewed each time the auditors are changed.

5.4.5 How should the committee review external audit assignment reports?

External audit will issue a number of reports over the year, some of which are required under the *Codes of Audit Practice* and *International Standards on Auditing (UK and Ireland)*, while others will depend upon the contents of the agreed audit plan.

Before reviewing the findings of any report, the committee should ensure that the scope of the work is absolutely clear so that all committee members understand what has and (more importantly) what has not been included within the audit review. Initially, the committee should concentrate on the overall conclusion as this should indicate those issues that the external auditor wishes to draw to its attention.

Committee time should focus on the major findings along with an assurance that line management is dealing with the other (less significant) issues. The main question for the committee should be whether the findings are consistent with their own appreciation of the issues from other information received, either in the committee or as a governing body member. If they are inconsistent then committee members should probe further and challenge the findings.

The response of management to audit findings is vital. The committee should consider:

- Whether management has responded to the audit appropriately?
- Whether the report highlights issues relating to policies and processes, or with the people implementing them?
- Whether management has agreed a realistic and timely action plan to remedy any problems?
- When the action plan will be followed up by management and the external auditors?
- What further work is required to complete the audit?

> **External Audit Reports – Best Practice and Questions to Consider**
>
> - The audit committee will wish to establish that the report arising from each external audit assignment is issued to the organisation's management on a timely basis
> - Audit committees should receive regular reports arising from work planned by external audit summarising activity in the period. The reports should describe the major audit issues, and report outcomes against the audit plan

---

[5] For organisations with external auditors appointed by the Audit Commission, approval must also be sought from the Commission.

- The audit committee should monitor the implementation of agreed actions by a variety of means – the aim being to review whether important recommendations have been actioned by management and that either assurance levels have improved or risks reduced. In each case the committee will wish to consider whether to invite a relevant senior manager to report on progress
- The audit committee should discuss the conclusion reached on the arrangements to secure economy, efficiency and effectiveness in the use of resources, comparing the external auditors' assessment with committee members' own views and those of executive management
- The committee should ensure that external audit reports and audit recommendations are given due weight and attention.

5.4.6 How should the committee review external auditors' mandatory reports?

The main mandatory reports that audit committees receive from their external auditors are:

- A report to those charged with governance – prior to signing their audit report on the annual accounts, the auditor will issue this report to the audit committee setting out the findings from their audit. This is sometimes referred to as the ISA 260 report as it is a requirement under *International Standard on Auditing (UK & Ireland) 260*. The purpose of the report is to ensure that the governing body is aware of and has considered any issues arising from the audit before approving and adopting the annual report and accounts. Sometimes, the auditor will require a formal response from the governing body – for example, where there are errors in the accounts that have not been rectified by management, the auditor will ask the governing body to confirm that it agrees with management's decision not to make an amendment and give its reason
- A statutory report and opinion on the annual report and accounts
- A statutory conclusion on whether the audited body has made proper arrangements for securing economy, efficiency and effectiveness in its use of resources
- The annual audit letter.

In each case, the committee's role is to receive and review the reports.

In addition to these reports, the external auditors may issue:

- A Public Interest Report (PIR) – this is made where auditors consider a matter is sufficiently important to be brought to the attention of the audited body or public as a matter of urgency
- Referral to the Secretary of State (or Monitor) – this is made where it is believed that a decision has led to unlawful expenditure[6] or that an action is unlawful and likely to cause a loss.

Whenever a PIR is being considered the audit committee should receive a briefing from the external auditors on the statutory background and potential consequences. This should include

---

[6] 'Unlawful expenditure' includes a breach of the organisation's revenue or capital resource limit (where relevant).

the reasons why such a report is considered necessary and the steps taken to date by the auditors and the organisation. The committee should consider the contents of such a briefing and look in detail at the implications and necessary actions. In such instances, the issue should immediately be taken for consideration by the whole governing body.

5.5 How Does Clinical Audit Support the Audit Committee's Work?

The National Institute for Health and Care Excellence (NICE) and the Healthcare Quality Improvement Partnership (HQIP) define clinical audit as 'a quality improvement process that seeks to improve patient care and outcomes through systematic review of care against explicit criteria and the implementation of change'. It involves reviewing clinical performance and measuring that performance against agreed standards with the overall aim of refining clinical practice. As such, 'it is one of the key compliance tools at management's disposal and has an important role within the assurance agenda[7]'.

The components of clinical audit are:

- Setting standards
- Measuring current practice
- Comparing results with standards
- Changing the way things are done
- Re-auditing to make sure practice has improved.

For NHS governing bodies and audit committees, managing clinical risk is as important as managing financial and business risk and good clinical audit is, therefore, an enormous asset and source of assurance.

Clinical Audit: a Simple Guide for NHS Governing Bodies, published by HQIP, sets out twelve criteria for good local clinical audit:

Criteria for Good Local Clinical Audit

1. Clinical audit should be part of a structured programme.
2. Topics chosen should in the main be high risk, high volume or high cost or reflect national clinical audits, national service frameworks or NICE guidance.
3. Service users should be part of the clinical audit process.
4. Should be multidisciplinary in nature.
5. Clinical audit should include assessment of process and outcome of care.
6. Standards should be derived from good quality guidelines.
7. The sample size chosen should be adequate to produce credible results.
8. Managers should be actively involved in clinical audit and in particular in the development of action plans from clinical audit enquiry.
9. Action plans should address the local barriers to change and identify those responsible for service improvement.

---

[7] *Taking it on Trust,* Audit Commission, 2009.

10. Re-audit should be applied to ascertain whether improvements in care have been implemented as a result of clinical audit.
11. Systems, structures and specific mechanisms should be made available to monitor service improvements once the clinical audit cycle has been completed.
12. Each clinical audit should have a local lead.

The audit committee can provide the governing body with assurance concerning these criteria. For example, by seeking to understand:

- How the programme of clinical audit work is decided upon
- Whether the programme is at an appropriate level and reflects the organisation's strategic objectives
- The rigour of the processes in place for conducting clinical audits
- Whether all clinical audits are reported, in what form and to whom
- How matters arising are dealt with and followed up.

The audit committee should expect to see regular reports on the outcomes of clinical audit work and should invite to its meetings senior managers responsible for planning and delivering clinical audits. Historically, clinical audit processes have not been designed to provide the organisation with assurance on a risk based approach to clinical practices. The audit committee will therefore wish to consider, with the clinical governance (or other relevant) committee, how best to engage with clinical audit to meet its own need for assurances.

Case Study – an Internal Audit Review of Clinical Audit

Recognising the need to gain assurance on the systems in place to support high quality clinical care, a number of NHS audit committees have incorporated a review of the organisation's clinical audit system into their internal audit plans.

Clinical audit is one of the main components of clinical governance and is a central mechanism for reviewing clinical practice against extant standards, guidelines, policies and procedures. Effective clinical audit programmes enable staff to critically (and routinely) review how care is provided, to make changes in their practice and demonstrate (through re-audit) improvements in care quality. As part of local arrangements for high quality care, all NHS organisations are required to have in place a comprehensive programme of service improvement activities that includes clinicians and other professional staff participating in regular clinical audit and clinical audit is a core component of professional codes of practice. The need for all trusts to ensure that their clinical audit systems are robust has been highlighted in a number of reports over recent years, reinforcing the need for all health professionals to engage in regular clinical audit activity as part of their continuing professional development.

The role of clinical audit is a key component of good governance. It is essential therefore, that all organisations are able to evidence that their clinical audit system is robust, reflects both national and local priorities, is comprehensive and embedded across all clinical teams, with the outcomes from audit used to drive improvement and to enhance the overall quality of clinical care.

When thinking about working arrangements between internal and clinical audit, the Department of Health's joint protocol for internal and clinical audit is a useful source of reference – it is available on the archived pages of the Department's website[8] and provides guidance for internal auditors on working with clinical audit when assessing the clinical governance aspects of the assurance framework underpinning the governance statement.

5.6 How Does Counter (or Anti-) Fraud Activity Support the Audit Committee's Work?

The emphasis on dealing with fraud and corruption in the NHS has increased significantly over recent years and as a result, both counter fraud activities and security in the NHS are now overseen by NHS Protect (part of the NHS Business Services Authority).

NHS Protect's role is to lead on identifying and tackling crime across the NHS and the NHS standard contract requires provider organisations to put in place and maintain adequate counter fraud and security arrangements. Within one month of service commencement, the provider must complete the 'organisation crime profile' (effectively a crime risk assessment) using the relevant toolkit provided by NHS Protect and in accordance with NHS guidance. Following its completion, the provider must take the necessary action to meet the standards set by NHS Protect at the level indicated by the completed crime profile. These standards cover:

- Strategic governance
- Inform and involve
- Prevent and deter
- Hold to account.

The NHS Protect quality assurance programme comprises two main processes that are closely linked to the standards:

- A quality assurance process that includes an annual self-review against the standards conducted by the organisation and submitted to NHS Protect with the annual report
- An assessment process conducted by NHS Protect's quality and compliance team in partnership with the organisation.

On the commissioning side, all CCGs are required to have access to 'appropriate, accredited counter fraud support' with the *Clinical Commissioning Group Guide for Applicants*, stating in criterion 4.2 that CCGs must be able to deliver all their statutory functions including strategic oversight, quality improvement, financial control and probity. CCGs are therefore expected to co-operate with NHS Protect and its nominated officers in the discharge of its functions – for example, by allowing NHS Protect access to CCG premises, members, employees, documents and information.

---

[8] *Joint Protocol for Internal Audit and Clinical Audit*, Department of Health, 2007:
http://webarchive.nationalarchives.gov.uk/+/www.dh.gov.uk/en/Managingyourorganisation/Workforce/Leadership/Governance/DH_4110194

The audit committee will wish to be aware of these NHS Protect requirements and satisfy itself that adequate arrangements are in place to ensure that they are met. The Committee will also want to consider the results of counter fraud and security work in so far as they have a bearing on the wider role of the committee. This means that work plans and reports about counter fraud and security activity will come to the audit committee so that it can:

- Assure itself that the plans give adequate coverage
- Consider the implications of the findings in the light of its wider knowledge of the organisation.

Counter fraud specialists will attend audit committee meetings at last twice a year and representatives from NHS Protect may also be invited on occasion.

> **Review of Counter Fraud and Security – Questions to Consider**
> - How is the scope of counter fraud and security work decided?
> - Are any scope restrictions placed on counter fraud and security activity and, if so, who establishes them?
> - Is counter fraud activity (including outcomes from the NHS Protect quality assurance programme) reported directly to an appropriate level of management that will ensure that counter fraud work is given due weight and attention?
> - Are those working on counter fraud and security activity free from any operational responsibilities that could impair their objectivity?
> - Do those working on counter fraud and security activity have a right of direct access to the audit committee Chair?
> - Is the technical knowledge and experience of those working on counter fraud and security activity sufficient to ensure that duties are performed to an appropriate standard?

5.7 What is the Audit Committee's Role in Relation to Whistle Blowing?

As mentioned in 1.6, the committee has a role in reviewing the effectiveness of the arrangements by which staff may raise concerns in confidence about possible improprieties relating to financial, clinical or organisational matters. The Financial Reporting Council's *Guidance on Audit Committees* suggests that the audit committee's aim in this area is to 'ensure that arrangements are in place for the proportionate and independent investigation of such matters and for appropriate follow-up action.' Monitor's *Code of Governance* (provision C.3.8) also emphasises that it is the role of the audit committee to review whistle blowing arrangements.

It is important to bear in mind that this does not mean that the audit committee looks into the detail of every reported incident.

5.8 What is the Value of Private Discussions with the Auditors?

Private discussions between audit committee members and each of the sets of auditors (and counter fraud specialists), without management present, is an important part of building up a relationship of trust and supporting the independence of the audit functions. These discussions should be formally scheduled and will generally take place before at least one meeting a year. In terms of approach, meetings can use a standard set of questions (see below) or cover specific issues.

The value of these discussions is to allow committee members and the auditors freedom to discuss a range of matters, without any perceived or actual management influence. They also provide an opportunity for the auditors to feedback to the audit committee on their own performance. These discussions should not be minuted, unless both the committee and auditors agree that a record would be pertinent. If this is the case, a note could be added to the committee's minutes. The Chair of the committee may wish to retain his/her own note of the discussion.

Non-executive directors/lay members on the audit committee may also wish to meet from time to time without others present.

> **Private Discussions with Auditors – Questions to Consider**
>
> - Do the internal auditors have adequate resources to provide the assurances required by the audit committee?
> - Have the external auditors quoted for enough resources to meet their statutory functions?
> - Did the auditors receive all the cooperation they needed?
> - Was any attempt made to restrict the scope of the auditors' work in any way?
> - Was the original audit strategy or plan modified due to deficiencies in internal control or accounting records?
> - Did the auditors have any significant disagreements with management? If so, how were these resolved?
> - Do the auditors have any concerns about management's control consciousness or operating style?
> - What is the auditors' view of their relationship with management?
> - Do the auditors believe they are under any undue pressure to give a particular opinion?
> - Do the auditors believe management are under undue pressure – for example, to report performance in a particular way?
> - Are there any other matters that, in the opinion of the auditors, should be considered by the audit committee?
> - Do the auditors have any comments on the way the audit committee operates and its effectiveness?

Appendix A: Example Terms of Reference

> These terms of reference reflect the particular nature of audit committees in the NHS and their role in developing integrated governance arrangements and providing assurance that NHS bodies are well managed across the whole range of their activities. They are designed to be generic and draw on existing terms of reference in use in a number of organisations. They are also consistent with NHS England's template for CCG audit committees.[1]

Terms of Reference

Constitution

The governing body hereby resolves to establish a committee of the governing body to be known as the audit committee (the Committee). The Committee is a non-executive committee of the governing body and has no executive powers, other than those specifically delegated in these terms of reference.

Membership

The Committee shall be appointed by the governing body from amongst its independent, non-executive directors/lay members and shall consist of not less than three members. A quorum shall be two of the three independent members. One of the members will be appointed Chair of the Committee[2] by the governing body. The Chair of the organisation itself shall not be a member of the Committee.

Attendance at meetings

The Chief Finance Officer and appropriate internal and external audit representatives shall normally attend meetings.

The counter fraud specialist will attend a minimum of two committee meetings a year.

The Accountable (or Accounting Officer) should be invited to attend meetings and should discuss at least annually with the audit committee the process for assurance that supports the governance statement. He or she should also attend when the Committee considers the draft annual governance statement and the annual report and accounts.

Other executive directors/managers should be invited to attend, particularly when the Committee is discussing areas of risk or operation that are the responsibility of that director/manager.

Representatives from other organisations (for example, NHS Protect) and other individuals[3] may be invited to attend on occasion.

---

[1] *CCG Governing Body Audit Committee Terms of Reference*, NHS England, 2012: www.england.nhs.uk/resources/resources-for-ccgs/ccg-tor/
[2] In CCGs, the Chair will be the lay member for governance.
[3] In CCGs, the governing body Chair may be invited to attend one meeting a year so that they can understand how the committee works.

The organisation's secretary (or governance lead) shall be secretary to the Committee and shall attend to take minutes of the meeting and provide appropriate support to the Chair and committee members.

At least once a year the Committee should meet privately with the external and internal auditors.

Access

The Head of Internal Audit, representative of external audit and counter fraud specialist have a right of direct access to the Chair of the committee.

Frequency of meetings

The Committee must consider the frequency and timing of meetings needed to allow it to discharge all of its responsibilities. A benchmark of five meetings per annum at appropriate times in the reporting and audit cycle is suggested. The governing body, Accounting (or Accountable) Officer, external auditors or Head of Internal Audit may request an additional meeting if they consider that one is necessary.

Authority

The Committee is authorised by the governing body to investigate any activity within its terms of reference. It is authorised to seek any information it requires from any employee and all employees are directed to cooperate with any request made by the Committee. The Committee is authorised by the governing body to obtain outside legal or other independent professional advice and to secure the attendance of outsiders with relevant experience and expertise if it considers this necessary.

Responsibilities

The Committee's duties/responsibilities can be categorised as follows:

Integrated governance, risk management and internal control

The Committee shall review the establishment and maintenance of an effective system of integrated governance, risk management and internal control, across the whole of the organisation's activities (clinical and non-clinical), that supports the achievement of the organisation's objectives.

In particular, the Committee will review the adequacy and effectiveness of:

- All risk and control related disclosure statements (in particular the governance statement), together with any accompanying Head of Internal Audit Opinion, external audit opinion or other appropriate independent assurances, prior to submission to the governing body
- The underlying assurance processes that indicate the degree of achievement of the organisation's objectives, the effectiveness of the management of principal risks and the appropriateness of the above disclosure statements

- The policies for ensuring compliance with relevant regulatory, legal and code of conduct requirements and any related reporting and self-certifications
- The policies and procedures for all work related to counter fraud and security as required by NHS Protect.

In carrying out this work the Committee will primarily utilise the work of internal audit, external audit and other assurance functions, but will not be limited to these sources. It will also seek reports and assurances from directors and managers as appropriate, concentrating on the over-arching systems of integrated governance, risk management and internal control, together with indicators of their effectiveness.

This will be evidenced through the Committee's use of an effective assurance framework to guide its work and the audit and assurance functions that report to it.

As part of its integrated approach, the Committee will have effective relationships with other key committees (for example, the quality committee) so that it understands processes and linkages. However, these other committees must not usurp the Committee's role.

Internal audit

The Committee shall ensure that there is an effective internal audit function that meets the *Public Sector Internal Audit Standards, 2013*[4] and provides appropriate independent assurance to the Committee, Accountable (or Accounting) Officer and governing body. This will be achieved by:

- Considering the provision of the internal audit service and the costs involved
- Reviewing and approving the annual internal audit plan and more detailed programme of work, ensuring that this is consistent with the audit needs of the organisation as identified in the assurance framework
- Considering the major findings of internal audit work (and management's response), and ensuring coordination between the internal and external auditors to optimise the use of audit resources
- Ensuring that the internal audit function is adequately resourced and has appropriate standing within the organisation
- Monitoring the effectiveness of internal audit and carrying out an annual review.

External audit

The Committee shall review and monitor the external auditors' independence and objectivity and the effectiveness of the audit process. In particular, the Committee will review the work and findings of the external auditors and consider the implications and management's responses to their work. This will be achieved by:

---

[4] These standards apply to all non-foundation NHS trusts and CCGs. Although they are not mandatory for FTs, Monitor has bought them to FTs' attention.

- Considering the appointment and performance of the external auditors, as far as the rules governing the appointment permit (and make recommendations to the governing body when appropriate)
- Discussing and agreeing with the external auditors, before the audit commences, the nature and scope of the audit as set out in the annual plan
- Discussing with the external auditors their evaluation of audit risks and assessment of the organisation and the impact on the audit fee
- Reviewing all external audit reports, including the report to those charged with governance (before its submission to the governing body) and any work undertaken outside the annual audit plan, together with the appropriateness of management responses
- Ensuring that there is in place a clear policy for the engagement of external auditors to supply non audit services.

Other assurance functions

The Committee shall review the findings of other significant assurance functions, both internal and external to the organisation, and consider the implications for the governance of the organisation.

These will include, but will not be limited to, any reviews by Department of Health arm's length bodies or regulators/inspectors (for example, the Care Quality Commission, NHS Litigation Authority, etc.) and professional bodies with responsibility for the performance of staff or functions (for example, Royal Colleges, accreditation bodies, etc.)

In addition, the Committee will review the work of other committees within the organisation, whose work can provide relevant assurance to the Committee's own areas of responsibility. In particular, this will include any clinical governance, risk management or quality committees that are established.

In reviewing the work of a clinical governance committee, and issues around clinical risk management, the Committee will wish to satisfy itself on the assurance that can be gained from the clinical audit function.

Counter fraud

The Committee shall satisfy itself that the organisation has adequate arrangements in place for counter fraud and security that meet NHS Protect's standards and shall review the outcomes of work in these areas.

Management

The Committee shall request and review reports, evidence and assurances from directors and managers on the overall arrangements for governance, risk management and internal control.

The Committee may also request specific reports from individual functions within the organisation (for example, clinical audit).

Financial reporting

The Committee shall monitor the integrity of the financial statements of the organisation and any formal announcements relating to its financial performance.

The Committee should ensure that the systems for financial reporting to the governing body, including those of budgetary control, are subject to review as to the completeness and accuracy of the information provided.

The Committee shall review the annual report and financial statements before submission to the governing body, focusing particularly on:

- The wording in the annual governance statement and other disclosures relevant to the terms of reference of the Committee
- Changes in, and compliance with, accounting policies, practices and estimation techniques
- Unadjusted mis-statements in the financial statements
- Significant judgements in preparation of the financial statements
- Significant adjustments resulting from the audit
- Letters of representation
- Explanations for significant variances.

Whistle blowing

The Committee shall review the effectiveness of the arrangements in place for allowing staff to raise (in confidence) concerns about possible improprieties in financial, clinical or safety matters and ensure that any such concerns are investigated proportionately and independently.

Reporting

The Committee shall report to the governing body on how it discharges its responsibilities.

The minutes of the Committee's meetings shall be formally recorded by the secretary and submitted to the governing body. The Chair of the Committee shall draw to the attention of the governing body any issues that require disclosure to the full governing body, or require executive action.

The Committee will report to the governing body at least annually on its work in support of the annual governance statement, specifically commenting on:

- The fitness for purpose of the assurance framework
- The completeness and 'embeddedness' of risk management in the organisation
- The integration of governance arrangements
- The appropriateness of the evidence that shows the organisation is fulfilling regulatory requirements relating to its existence as a functioning business
- The robustness of the processes behind the quality accounts.

This annual report should also describe how the Committee has fulfilled its terms of reference and give details of any significant issues that the Committee considered in relation to the financial statements and how they were addressed.

Administrative support

The Committee shall be supported administratively by its secretary (the organisation's secretary or governance lead) – his or her duties in this respect will include:

- Agreement of agendas with the Chair and attendees
- Preparation, collation and circulation of papers in good time
- Ensuring that those invited to each meeting attend
- Taking the minutes and helping the Chair to prepare reports to the governing body
- Keeping a record of matters arising and issues to be carried forward
- Arranging meetings for the Chair – for example, with the internal/external auditors or local counter fraud specialists
- Maintaining records of members' appointments and renewal dates etc
- Advising the Committee on pertinent issues/areas of interest/policy developments
- Ensuring that action points are taken forward between meetings
- Ensuring that Committee members receive the development and training they need.

Appendix B: Example Agenda and Timetable

This appendix assumes that an audit committee meets five times each year and gives an indication of when key items are likely to appear on the agenda.

Agenda item/Issue	1 March	2 May	3 July	4 Sept/Oct	5 Jan
Governance					
Review the assurance framework			X		X
Review the risk management system					X
Note business of other committees and review inter-relationships	X		X	X	X
Review draft annual governance statement	X	X			
Receive other sources of assurance	X		X	X	X
Review the annual report and accounts			X		
Review the quality account/report			X		
Review whistle blowing arrangements				X	
Review other reports and policies as appropriate – for example, changes to standing orders		X			X
Financial focus					
Agree final annual report and accounts timetable and plans				X	
Review annual report and accounts progress	X				
Review audited annual accounts and financial statements (including the external audit opinion)		X			
Review risks and controls around financial management			X		X
Review changes to standing orders, standing financial instructions/prime financial policies and changes to accounting policies	X		X		X
Review losses and special payments	X	X	X	X	X
Internal audit					
Review and approve annual internal audit plan	X				
Review and approve internal audit terms of reference	X				
Annual review of the effectiveness of internal audit					X
Review internal audit progress reports	X		X	X	X

Example Agenda and Timetable

Agenda item/Issue	1 March	2 May	3 July	4 Sept/Oct	5 Jan
Receive annual internal audit report and associated opinions	×	×			
External audit					
Agree external audit plans and fees	×				×
Review the effectiveness of external audit				×	
Review external audit progress reports	×	×	×	×	×
Receive the external auditor's report to those charged with governance			×		
Receive/consider the external auditor's annual audit letter				×	
Clinical audit (if applicable)					
Review annual clinical audit plan	×				
Review clinical audit terms of reference	×				
Review the effectiveness of clinical audit				×	
Review clinical audit progress reports	×		×	×	×
Counter fraud and security					
Review and approve the annual work plan for counter fraud and security activity	×				
Review counter fraud and security progress reports	×		×	×	×
Review the organisation's annual self-review against NHS Protect's standards		×			
Review the effectiveness of the those carrying out counter fraud and security activity					×
Receive the annual report on counter fraud and security activity		×			
Other activities					
Plan how to discharge the committee's duties	×				
Self-assess the committee's effectiveness					×
Review the committee's terms of reference				×	
Produce the annual committee report	×				
Private discussions with internal and external auditors (and counter fraud specialists)			×		
Briefing/update sessions		×		×	

Appendix C: Self-assessment Checklists

This appendix includes two checklists designed to help in assessing the effectiveness of the audit committee. The first focuses on committee administration; the second on how well the committee operates over a number of categories.

Checklist One: Committee Processes

This checklist is designed to elicit a simple yes or no answer to each question and could be completed by the Chair with the assistance of the committee's secretary. As it is closely linked to the terms of reference set out in appendix A, it is suggested that the results are reported to the audit committee. Where 'no' answers have been given, the issues should be debated at a committee meeting to determine if any further action is needed.

Area/Question	Yes	No	Comments/Action
Composition, establishment and duties			
Does the audit committee have written terms of reference that adequately define the committee's role in accordance with relevant guidance (for example from the Department of Health; NHS England; NHS Trust Development Authority or Monitor)?			
Have the terms of reference been adopted by the governing body?			
Are the terms of reference reviewed annually to take into account governance developments and the remit of other committees within the organisation?			
Are committee members independent of the management team?			
Are the outcomes of each meeting; the actions taken and the committee's view on the organisation's systems of internal control reported to the next governing body meeting?			
Does the committee prepare an annual report on its work and performance in the preceding year for consideration by the governing body?			
Does the committee assess its own effectiveness periodically?			
Has the committee established a plan of matters to be dealt with across the year?			
Are committee papers distributed in sufficient time for members to give them due consideration?			
Has the committee been quorate for each meeting this year?			

Self-assessment Checklists

Area/Question	Yes	No	Comments/Action
Compliance with the law and regulations governing the NHS			
Does the committee review assurance and regulatory compliance reporting processes?			
Does the committee have a mechanism to keep it aware of topical, legal and regulatory issues?			
Internal control and risk management			
Has the committee formally considered how it integrates with other committees that are reviewing risk – for example, risk management, quality and clinical governance committees?			
Has the committee reviewed the robustness and effectiveness of the content of the organisation's assurance framework?			
Has the committee reviewed the robustness and content of the draft annual governance statement before it is presented to the governing body?			
Is the committee's role in reviewing and recommending to the governing body the annual report and accounts clearly defined?			
Does the committee consider the external auditor's report to those charged with governance including proposed adjustments to the accounts?			
Internal audit			
Is there a formal 'charter' or terms of reference, defining internal audit's objectives, responsibilities and reporting lines?			
Does the committee review and approve the internal audit plan at the beginning of the financial year?			
Does the committee approve any material changes to the plan?			
Is the committee confident that the audit plan is derived from a clear risk assessment process that links closely to the assurance framework?			
Does the committee receive periodic progress reports from the Head of Internal Audit?			
Does the committee effectively monitor the implementation of management actions arising from internal audit reports?			
Does the Head of Internal Audit have a right of access to the committee and its Chair at any time?			

Area/Question	Yes	No	Comments/Action
Is the committee confident that internal audit is free of any scope restrictions and, if not, has it considered the impact of these on the annual Head of Internal Audit opinion?			
Is the committee confident that internal audit is free from any operational responsibilities or conflicts of interest that could impair its objectivity?			
Does the committee hold periodic private discussions with the Head of Internal Audit?			
Has the committee evaluated whether internal audit complies with the *Public Sector Internal Audit Standards*?			
Has the committee agreed a range of internal audit performance measures to be reported on a routine basis?			
Does the committee receive and review the Head of Internal Audit's annual opinion?			
External audit			
Do the external auditors present their audit plans and strategy to the committee for agreement and approval?			
Does the committee receive and monitor actions taken relating to prior years' reviews?			
Does the committee review the external auditor's ISA 260 report (the report to those charged with governance)?			
Does the committee review the external auditor's value for money conclusion?			
Does the committee review the external auditor's opinion on the quality account when necessary [Note: this question is not relevant for CCGs]			
Does the committee hold periodic private discussions with the external auditors?			
Does the committee assess the performance of external audit?			
Does the committee require assurance from external audit about its policies for ensuring independence?			
Has the committee approved a policy to govern the nature and value of non-audit work carried out by the external auditors?			
Does the committee receive information on all non-audit work undertaken by external audit?			
Does the committee review the proportion of audit and non-audit work every time the external auditors change?			

Self-assessment Checklists

Area/Question	Yes	No	Comments/Action
Clinical audit [Note: this section is only relevant for providers]			
Is the committee clear about where clinical audit assurances are received and monitored?			
If the committee is NOT the main committee receiving direct feedback from clinical audit, does it receive a report from the relevant committee on the progress made by clinical audit during the year along with a clear view on the outcome of the annual work plan?			
If the committee receives reports from clinical audit has it: • Reviewed an annual plan which is clearly linked to clinical risks and clinical assurance needs? • Received regular progress reports? • Monitored the implementation of management actions resulting from clinical audit reviews? • Received a report over the quality assurance processes covered by clinical audit activity?			
Counter (or anti-) fraud and security			
Is the committee aware of NHS Protect requirements in relation to counter fraud and security activity?			
Does the committee review the planned counter fraud and security work at the beginning of the financial year and in particular its scope and coverage?			
Does the committee satisfy itself that the work plan is derived from clear processes based on risk assessments and that coverage is adequate?			
Does the committee receive notification of any material changes to the plan?			
Does the committee receive periodic reports about counter fraud and security activity?			
Does the committee effectively monitor the implementation of management actions arising from counter fraud and security reports?			
Do those working on counter fraud and security activity have a right of direct access to the committee and its Chair?			
Do those working on counter fraud and security activity have the necessary technical knowledge and experience to ensure that work is carried out as it should be?			
Does the committee receive and review an annual report on counter fraud and security activity?			

Area/Question	Yes	No	Comments/Action
Does the committee receive and discuss reports arising from inspections by NHS Protect in relation to the quality of the counter fraud (and security) provision?			
Annual report and accounts and disclosure statements			
Is the committee's role in the approval of the annual report and accounts clearly defined?			
Is a committee meeting scheduled to discuss proposed adjustments to the accounts and issues arising from the audit?			
Does the committee specifically review: • Changes in accounting policies? • Changes in accounting practice due to changes in accounting standards? • Changes in estimation techniques? • Significant judgements made in preparing the accounts? • Significant adjustments resulting from the audit? • Explanations for any significant variances?			
Does the committee ensure it receives explanations for any unadjusted errors in the accounts found by the external auditors?			
Does the committee receive and review a draft of the organisation's annual governance statement?			
Does the committee receive and review a draft of the organisation's annual report and accounts?			
Does the committee receive and review the evidence required to demonstrate compliance with regulatory requirements (for example, as set by the Care Quality Commission, Monitor and the NHS Trust Development Authority)?			
Other issues			
Does the committee provide a summary report of its meetings to the next available governing body meeting?			
Has the committee reviewed its performance in the year for consistency with its: • Terms of reference? • Programme for the year?			

Self-assessment Checklists

Checklist Two: Committee Effectiveness

This checklist is designed to gauge the committee's effectiveness by taking the views of committee members across a number of themes. It is suggested that every member of the audit committee completes the checklist and the Chair and secretary review the results and use their judgement to recommend any further actions required. Alternatively, the committee may decide to work through the checklist collectively.

Statement	Strongly agree	Agree	Disagree	Strongly disagree	Unable to answer	Comments/ action
Theme 1 – committee focus						
The committee has set itself a series of objectives it wants to achieve this year.						
The committee has made a conscious decision about how it wants to operate in terms of the level of information it would like to receive for each of the items on its cycle of business.						
Committee members contribute regularly across the range of issues discussed.						
The committee is fully aware of the key sources of assurance and who provides them in support of the controls mitigating the key risks to the organisation.						
The committee clearly understands and receives assurances from third parties the organisation uses to manage/ operate key functions – for example, financial services operated by NHS Shared Business Services, other NHS bodies, commissioning support units or private contractors.						
Equal prominence is given to both quality and financial assurance.						
Theme 2 – committee team working						
The committee has the right balance of experience, knowledge and skills to fulfil the role described in the *NHS Audit Committee Handbook*.						

Statement	Strongly agree	Agree	Disagree	Strongly disagree	Unable to answer	Comments/ action
The committee has structured its agenda to cover, quality, data quality, performance targets and financial control.						
The committee ensures that the relevant executive director/manager attends meetings to enable it to secure the required level of understanding of the reports and information it receives (i.e. the right executive lead is there to discuss risk and internal matters in their area of responsibility rather than the committee having to rely on the CFO to act as conduit to the executive team).						
Management fully briefs the committee via the assurance framework in relation to the key risks and assurances received and any gaps in control/ assurance in a timely fashion thereby eradicating the potential for 'surprises'.						
Other committees provide timely and clear information in support of the committee thereby eradicating the potential for 'surprises'.						
I feel sufficiently comfortable within the committee environment to be able to express my views, doubts and opinions.						
I understand the messages being given by the organisation's assurance advisors (external audit/internal audit/counter fraud specialists).						
Internal audit contributes to the debate across the range of the agenda and not just on the papers they present.						

Self-assessment Checklists

Statement	Strongly agree	Agree	Disagree	Strongly disagree	Unable to answer	Comments/ action
Members hold their assurance providers to account for late or missing assurances.						
When a decision has been made or action agreed I feel confident that it will be implemented as agreed and in line with the timescale set down.						
Theme 3 – committee effectiveness						
The quality of committee papers received allows me to perform my role effectively.						
Members provide real and genuine challenge – they do not just seek clarification and/or reassurance.						
Debate is allowed to flow and conclusions reached without being cut short or stifled due to time constraints etc.						
Each agenda item is 'closed off' appropriately so that I am clear what the conclusion is; who is doing what, when and how etc and how it is being monitored.						
At the end of each meeting we discuss the outcomes and reflect back on decisions made and what worked well, not so well etc.						
The committee provides a written summary report of its meetings to the governing body.						
The governing body challenges and understands the reporting from this committee.						
There is a formal appraisal of the committee's effectiveness each year which is evidence based and takes into account my views and external views.						

Statement	Strongly agree	Agree	Disagree	Strongly disagree	Unable to answer	Comments/ action
Theme 4 – committee engagement						
The committee actively challenges both management and other assurance providers during the year to gain a clear understanding of their findings.						
The committee is clear about the complementary relationship it has with other governing body committees that play a role in relation to clinical governance, quality and risk management.						
The committee receives clear and timely reports from other governing body committees which set out the assurances they have received and their impact (either positive or not) on the organisation's assurance framework.						
I can provide two examples of where we as a committee have focused on improvements to the system of internal control as a result of assurance gaps identified.						
Theme 5 – committee leadership						
The committee Chair has a positive impact on the performance of the committee.						
Committee meetings are chaired effectively and with clarity of purpose and outcome.						
The committee Chair is visible within the organisation and is considered approachable.						
The committee Chair allows debate to flow freely and does not assert his/her own views too strongly.						
The committee Chair provides clear and concise information to the governing body on the activities of the committee and the implications of all identified gaps in assurance/control.						

Appendix D: Internal Audit Coverage

> One of the key sources of assurance relied on by audit committees to help them discharge their duties is an effective internal audit function. As we have seen in section 5.3.1, professional standards require that internal audit planning is driven by an assessment of the needs of each organisation based on its individual risk profile and assurance framework. The aim of this appendix is to give a more detailed indication of the range of activities that an internal audit plan may include for both a provider and commissioning organisation.

Please note that, when looking through the lists that follow, it is important to bear in mind that they are not intended to be exhaustive and should not be used as a checklist against which to compare internal audit's annual plan. Instead they are designed to give audit committees an idea of the issues that may crop up in their discussions with internal auditors when the annual plan is being considered.

> **Example One: NHS Provider Organisation**
>
> **Governance**
> Risk management and assurance framework
> Corporate governance/integrated governance
> Clinical governance framework/Monitor's quality governance framework
> Partnership working, joint ventures and subsidiaries (including hosted services)
> Regulatory compliance/returns
> Engagement with patients and public/marketing and communication strategy
> Standards of business conduct – for example, managing conflicts of interest, whistleblowing
> Complaints and claims management – handling/learning lessons
> Policy management/maintenance
> Management of projects and business cases
> Medical research and development governance
> Business continuity
> Freedom of information compliance
>
> **Clinical/patient safety**
> Clinical/safety monitoring and improvement systems
> Theatre safety
> Clinical audit
> Pharmacy, prescribing and medicines management, including controlled drugs
> Safeguarding (adults and children)
> Incident management/serious incidents
> Patient consent
> Infection control
> Decontamination
> Medical devices/medical gases
> Emergency planning
> Food and nutrition
> Ward rostering/safe medical staffing

Clinical coding/clinical records/patients activity data capture, accuracy and integrity
Safety alert systems
Compliance with Mental Health Act
Ward/unit/site compliance visits – for example, mental health, prison and community care units

Quality/performance
Monitoring Care Quality Commission/National Institute for Health and Care Excellence (NICE) compliance
Third party assessments – for example, by the NHSLA
Quality accounts
Performance monitoring/management
Performance/board reporting – financial and quality (including early warning/key performance indicators)
QIPP (Quality, Innovation, Productivity and Prevention)
Care pathways – for example, the 18 week wait, ambulance handovers
Outpatient clinics and appointment process
Cancelled operations/DNA management
Referral/demand management – for example, A&E/inappropriate non-emergency admissions
Discharge and bed management/delayed transfers of care
Patient experience – for example, the friends and family test
Benchmarking/VFM/consultancy reviews

Financial control
Financial accounting/general ledger
Budgetary control/management reporting
Income and debtor accounting
Expenditure and creditor accounting
Capital accounting
Payroll controls
Cost improvement programme/financial recovery and turnaround plans
Procurement and contract management including tender/waivers compliance
Treasury/cash flow management
Charitable funds
Private patients/fee-paying patients – for example, overseas
Losses and compensation payments
Patients monies and property

Information management and technology
Information governance
IT strategy
IT security – system/network/pc/applications
Disaster recovery/data security
Data quality
System/application controls – for example, pathology, choose and book

New system/application implementation projects
Desktop/PC maintenance/support services
Monitoring/management of IT service level agreement
Data protection act compliance
Firewall controls
Data leakage
Encryption
Mobile device management

Human resources
HR systems and ESR (electronic staff record) including recruitment/professional registration checks
Workforce management and planning/organisational development and retention strategy
Statutory and essential/mandatory training
Appraisals and clinical supervision
Doctor revalidation
Consultants job planning
Use of interims/consultancy
Bank and agency staffing/use of locums
Absence management
Leaver controls/management of salary overpayments
Time and attendance systems – for example, e-rostering, working time directive

Estates and facilities
Capital planning, monitoring and projects
Estates and equipment maintenance (planned, preventative and reactive)
Sustainability/carbon reduction strategy
Asset management – for example, theatre utilisation, stores/stock/community equipment
Security management
Health and safety including fire safety
Other FM services – for example, catering, parking, cleaning, waste, grounds, porters, laundry, post and telecoms

Example Two: Clinical Commissioning Group

Governance
Risk management and assurance framework
Corporate governance/integrated governance
Clinical governance framework
Partnership working – for example, health and wellbeing boards
Member practice engagement
Engagement with patients/public
Managing conflicts of interest
Complaints management – handling/learning lessons
Emergency planning and business continuity

Clinical/patient safety
  Clinical/safety monitoring and improvement systems
  Prescribing and medicines management
  Safeguarding (adults and children)
  Serious incidents
  Continuing healthcare and funded nursing care
  Clinical audit
  Compliance with Mental Health Act (s136, placements etc.)

Quality/performance
  Performance monitoring/management
  Performance reporting – financial and quality
  Monitoring Care Quality Commission/NICE compliance
  Third party assessments – for example by the NHSLA/CQC
  QIPP (Quality, Innovation, Productivity and Prevention)
  Benchmarking/VFM/consultancy reviews
  Collaborative arrangements with commissioning support units

Commissioning, procurement and contract management
  Clinical commissioning cycle – commissioning, monitoring and SLA management
  Specific clinical procurement – for example, local enhanced services, out of hours etc.
  Commissioning improvements/care pathway redesign
  Monitoring provider/patient services cost/quality – for example, care homes
  Referral/demand management – for example, A&E/inappropriate non-emergency admissions
  Joint risk pools/management of contingency
  Non-clinical procurement – for example, tendering and contracting
  Contract management/development of the commissioning support unit
  Continuing healthcare

Financial control
  Financial accounting/general ledger
  Budgetary control/management reporting
  Income and debtor accounting
  Expenditure and creditor accounting
  Capital accounting
  Payroll controls
  GP payments
  Direct payments
  Individual funding requests

Information management and technology
  Information governance
  IT strategy
  IT security – system/network/pc/applications
  Disaster recovery/data security

Data quality
System/application controls – for example, pathology and choose and book etc.
New system/application implementation projects
Desktop/PC maintenance/support services
Monitoring/management of IT service level agreement
Data Protection Act compliance
Firewall controls
Data leakage
Encryption
Mobile device management

Human resources
HR systems (recruitment/retention)
Statutory/mandatory training, appraisals and supervision
Use of consultants/interim staff
Absence management
Leaver controls
Management of overpayments
Workforce planning
Organisational development

Appendix E: References and Further Reading

UK Corporate Governance Code, Financial Reporting Council, 2012:
https://www.frc.org.uk/Our-Work/Codes-Standards/Corporate-governance/UK-Corporate-Governance-Code.aspx

Guidance on Audit Committees, Financial Reporting Council, 2012:
https://www.frc.org.uk/Our-Work/Publications/Corporate-Governance/Guidance-on-Audit-Committees-September-2012.aspx

Audit and Risk Assurance Committee Handbook, HM Treasury, 2013:
https://www.gov.uk/government/publications/audit-committee-handbook

The NHS Foundation Trust Code of Governance, Monitor, 2013:
www.monitor.gov.uk/FTcode

Audit Code for NHS Foundation Trusts, Monitor, 2011:
http://www.monitor-nhsft.gov.uk/home/our-publications/browse-category/guidance-foundation-trusts/mandatory-guidance/audit-code-nhs-f

NHS Wales Audit Committee Handbook, 2012:
www.wales.nhs.uk/governance-emanual/document/213861

NHS Act 2006: www.legislation.gov.uk/ukpga/2006/41/contents

Model Constitution Framework for Clinical Commissioning Groups, NHS England, 2012:
www.england.nhs.uk/resources/resources-for-ccgs/ccg-mod-cons-framework/

Code of Conduct and Accountability, NHS Trust Development Authority, 2013:
www.ntda.nhs.uk/wp-content/uploads/2013/04/CODE-OF-CONDUCT-AND-ACCOUNTABILITY-FOR-NHS-BOARDS.pdf

1990 Trust Membership and Procedure Regulations (SI 1990/2024):
www.legislation.gov.uk/uksi/1990/2024/contents/made

The Orange Book: Management of Risk – Principles and Concepts, HM Treasury, 2004:
https://www.gov.uk/government/uploads/system/uploads/attachment_data/file/220647/orange_book.pdf

The Mid Staffordshire NHS Foundation Trust Public Inquiry:
www.midstaffspublicinquiry.com/

Care Quality Commission: www.cqc.org.uk/

Taking it On Trust, Audit Commission, 2009 (archived pages):
http://archive.audit-commission.gov.uk/auditcommission/nationalstudies/health/financialmanagement/Pages/takingitontrust29april2009.aspx.html

References and Further Reading

Health and Social Care Act 2012:
www.legislation.gov.uk/ukpga/2012/7/contents/enacted/data.htm

Health Service Bodies Audit Committees (consultation and latest position), Department of Health, 2013: https://www.gov.uk/government/consultations/new-requirements-for-nhs-audit-committees

Committee on Standards in Public Life (for details of the 'Nolan principles'):
http://www.public-standards.gov.uk/

CCG Governing Body Members: Role Outlines, Attributes and Skills, NHS England, 2012:
www.england.nhs.uk/wp-content/uploads/2012/09/ccg-members-roles.pdf

International Standard on Auditing (UK and Ireland) 260 – Communication with Those Charged with Governance, Financial Reporting Council, 2012:
https://www.frc.org.uk/Our-Work/Publications/Audit-and-Assurance-Team/ISA-(UK-and-Ireland)-260-Revised-October-2012.pdf

Managing Public Money, HM Treasury, 2013:
https://www.gov.uk/government/publications/managing-public-money

Securing Sustainability – Planning Guidance for NHS Trust Boards 2014/15 – 2018/19, NHS Trust Development Authority, 2013: www.ntda.nhs.uk/blog/2013/12/23/planning-guidance/

Delivering High Quality Care for Patients: The Accountability Framework, NHS Trust Development Authority, 2013:
www.ntda.nhs.uk/blog/2013/05/03/delivering-high-quality-care-for-patients-the-accountabilty-framework-2/

Health Act 2009: www.legislation.gov.uk/ukpga/2009/21/contents

Information about quality accounts (including links to regulations and guidance):
www.nhs.uk/aboutNHSChoices/professionals/healthandcareprofessionals/quality-accounts/Pages/about-quality-accounts.aspx

Code of Audit Practice, Audit Commission:
http://www.audit-commission.gov.uk/audit-regime/codes-of-audit-practice/

Local Audit and Accountability Act 2014:
www.legislation.gov.uk/ukpga/2014/2/contents/enacted/data.htm

Public Sector Internal Auditing Standards, 2013:
https://www.gov.uk/government/publications/public-sector-internal-audit-standards

ISAE 3402: Assurance Reports on Controls at a Service Organization, IFAC:
www.ifac.org/publications-resources/staff-overview-international-standard-assurance-engagements-isae-3402-assuran

International Standard on Auditing (UK and Ireland) 610 – Using the Work of Internal Auditors, FRC (revised 2013):
https://www.frc.org.uk/Our-Work/Publications/Audit-and-Assurance-Team/ISA-(UK-and-Ireland)-610-June-2013.aspx

National Institute for Health and Care Excellence (NICE): www.nice.org.uk/

Healthcare Quality Improvement Partnership (HQIP):
www.hqip.org.uk/national-clinical-audits-for-inclusion-in-quality-accounts

Clinical Audit: A Simple Guide for NHS Governing Bodies, HQIP, 2010:
www.hqip.org.uk/assets/Guidance/HQIP-Clinical-Audit-Simple-Guide-online1.pdf

Joint Protocol for Internal Audit and Clinical Audit, Department of Health, 2007:
webarchive.nationalarchives.gov.uk/+/www.dh.gov.uk/en/Managingyourorganisation/Workforce/Leadership/Governance/DH_4110194

NHS Protect: www.nhsbsa.nhs.uk/Protect.aspx

Clinical Commissioning Group Guide for Applicants, NHS England, 2012:
www.england.nhs.uk/resources/resources-for-ccgs/auth/

Terms of reference for CCG audit committees, NHS England, 2012:
www.england.nhs.uk/resources/resources-for-ccgs/ccg-tor/